HEALTHCARE TECHNOLOGIES SERIES 22

Control of Prosthetic Hands

Control of Prosthetic Hands

Challenges and emerging avenues

Edited by
Kianoush Nazarpour

The Institution of Engineering and Technology

Published by The Institution of Engineering and Technology, London, United Kingdom

The Institution of Engineering and Technology is registered as a Charity in England & Wales (no. 211014) and Scotland (no. SC038698).

The Institution of Engineering and Technology
Michael Faraday House
Six Hills Way, Stevenage
Herts, SG1 2AY, United Kingdom

www.theiet.org

British Library Cataloguing in Publication Data
A catalogue record for this product is available from the British Library

ISBN 978-1-78561-984-7 (hardback)
ISBN 978-1-78561-985-4 (PDF)

Typeset in India by MPS Limited

Contents

About the editor

Kianoush Nazarpour holds a Readership in Biomedical AI at School of Informatics, The University of Edinburgh. His research is motivated by the potential of technology to restore function to individuals with disability. He has authored over 110 peer-reviewed articles in peer-reviewed journals and conferences, and his work has received many awards, including the UNESCO Netexplo 2018 award, for the "Hand that Sees" project with the citation "one of the most promising digital innovations with impact on society and business."

Chapter 1
Control of prosthetic hands

Kianoush Nazarpour[1], Agamemnon Krasoulis[2]
and Janne M. Hahne[3]

It is estimated that more than 1.5 million people live with an absence of upper limb [1]. Upper limb referrals are prevalent in highly skilled technicians, engineering, war veterans and generally younger and more active age groups for whom lifetime care can be remarkably expensive. Prosthetic hands can improve their quality of life dramatically through contributing to their dignity, independence and more effective inclusion in society. Many prosthetic hands in the market these days are highly sophisticated, offering individual finger movement and even movement of segments within a finger which resemble the natural arm and hand. Surveys on the use of prosthetic hands, however, reveal that 45% of the paediatric users and 26% of the adult users abandon their prosthesis with the primary reason being that upper limb prostheses do not provide enough function. Other reasons include users finding them uncomfortable and unsuitable for their needs or cumbersome.

Upper limb prostheses can be divided into two broad categories: *passive* or *cosmetic* prostheses, which only aim at restoring the physical appearance of a missing body part, and *active* prostheses, which also aim at partially restoring upper limb function, including reaching and grasping. Depending on the mode of operation, active prostheses can be sub-classified into two categories: *body powered* and *muscle controlled*, also called *myoelectric*.

Upper limb prosthetics can be further classified based on the mechanical design of the terminal device. Traditionally, functional designs were preferred, for example grippers and split hooks, which enable users to grasp objects and perform other activities of daily living. Such models typically support only one function, that is, hand opening and closing. In the last two decades, models inspired by human anatomy have become increasingly more popular. In addition to resembling natural limbs, multi-articulated hands comprise several motors, typically one for each digit, and often an additional motor controlling the rotation of the thumb.

Figure 1.1 shows a basic block diagram for the control of active prosthetic hands. Once a movement or grip is intended in the human brain, the neural command signals travel down the spinal cord and manifest in the form of a movement signal. The control

[1]The University of Edinbugrh, Edinburgh, UK
[2]Newcastle University, Newcastle upon Tyne, UK
[3]University Medical Center Göttingen, Göttingen, Germany

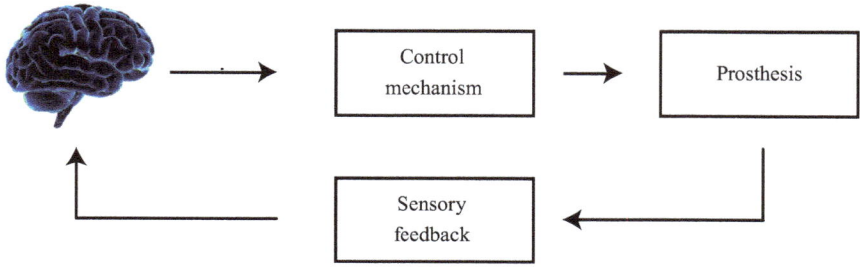

Figure 1.1   A block diagram for the control of prosthetic hands

unit in the prosthesis detects that activity and actuates the prosthesis. Feedback from the device, be it in the simple form of vision or otherwise, closes the control loop. Over decades, researchers and clinicians have invested a significant amount of resources in enhancing this control loop, both in the forward and in the feedback roots, from sensing movement intentions, enhancing the control mechanism, improving the terminal device and implementing effective ways of sensory feedback. Covering all these topics in-depth and discussing their subtleties and nuances in a book are impossible. But what we aim to achieve is to provide a current narrative as to how we see the research has evolved over the past years and share our vision as to where the field is aiming towards. This edited book has 11 chapters.

In this chapter, after this short introduction, we provide a review of the various methods for the control of active prosthetic hands. We introduce various conventional and contemporary approaches and lay the foundation of more advanced techniques that could achieve the holy grail of prosthesis control, that is, the continuous control of individual digits and wrist joints.

After the technical details that we present in the first chapter, we focus on the clinical aspects of prosthetic control in Chapters 2 and 3, namely, the design of bespoke sockets and clinical outcome measures, which are typically underappreciated by researchers who develop the controllers in the engineering and physical sciences domain. By bringing these two chapters in as early as possible in this book, we would like to promote the view that the likelihood of the translation of technical innovations is increased significantly if clinical expertise and outcome measures are considered from the outset.

Chapters 4–7 review the current state-of-the-art innovations that although currently are at low technology levels, they have the potential to revolutionalise the way prosthetic hands are controlled over the next decades. Specifically, we include methods that enable interfacing directly with the nerves and muscles and discuss current trends and future potentials. This section of the book is concluded by reviewing recent innovations in surgical techniques.

Chapter 8 reviews how artificial intelligence and machine learning have contributed to the field of prosthetic control. It then continues to define user-prosthesis co-adaptation and the challenges, technical and/or scientific, that need to be tackled to achieve a truly co-adaptive system. Finally, this chapter presents some current trends in machine learning that could enhance prosthetics control significantly.

Chapters 9 and 10 focus on another relatively understudied sub-field within prosthetics, that is, children prosthetics. Chapter 9 presents a broad overview of how the needs for prosthetics in children with limb difference (congenital and acquired) are different from adults and how new technologies can address these needs. It then discusses the use of methods based on 3D printing for children prosthetics and reviews the (limited) clinical evidence supporting their use. Chapter 10 then reports the fabrication and lab testing of a 3D-printed prosthesis, which is appropriate for children.

Finally, in Chapter 11, we conclude this book and share our vision of what the future could hold for the field of advanced prosthetics.

1.1 Prosthesis control types

1.1.1 Body powered

Before myoelectric prostheses were established, body-powered prostheses have been the most used technology for upper limb replacements. In fact, internationally, many people receive a body-powered prosthesis as their first prosthesis. Typically, the user can open or close the prosthesis by moving their contralateral shoulder and the force is picked up with a harness system and brought to the prosthesis with a Bowden cable (Figure 1.2). The established systems either actively close or open with contralateral shoulder motions, and the opposite movement is done with a spring in the prosthesis. There has been even a mechanical construction proposed that allows to switch between active closing and active opening. Although most prostheses in western countries today are electrically powered, the body-powered ones are still used and have also their advantages. They are relatively light, very robust and independent from power

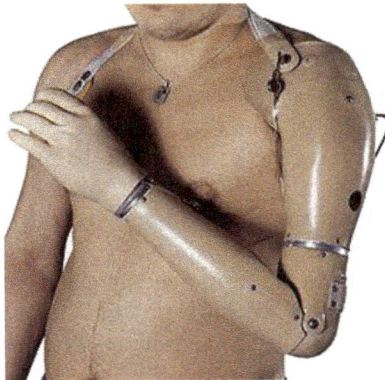

Figure 1.2 Body-powered prosthesis control. This figure is taken from the online source [2]

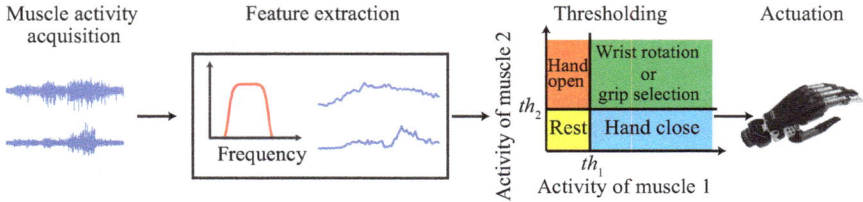

Muscle activity acquisition   Feature extraction   Thresholding   Actuation

Figure 1.3   Myocontrol with two sensors using the thresholding methods

supply. Also, they offer an intrinsic force feedback via the Bowden cable, which is not available in other prostheses.

1.1.2   Muscle control

The electromyographic (EMG) signal is the most important control source for electrically powered prostheses. It has been proposed by researchers after the Second World War [3], and the first commercial product was established in the 1960s in the USSR [4]. Typically active, bipolar electrode modules that integrate the amplification, filtering and envelope extraction are used. The short conduction path from the electrode contacts to the first amplification stage reduces the incoupling of external disturbances from the surrounding. Also the bipolar configuration leads to a significantly improved signal-to-noise ratio. Figure 1.3 summarises the control block diagram using the thresholding method. The route for sensory feedback is typically not available in current clinical systems and therefore not included in the figure.

1.2   Neurophysiology of movement

Voluntary motor control is the process by which living organisms coordinate their muscles in order to perform voluntary movement and actions. It involves the coordination of several subsystems of the central and peripheral nervous system, including primary and premotor cortical areas, the brainstem, basal ganglia, cerebellum and spinal cord circuits [5].

In healthy, able-bodied humans, all motions are conducted via muscle contractions that are initiated in the motor cortex of the brain. The commands for contractions are transferred from the cortex in the form of action potentials via efferent neurons through the spinal cord and nerves to the muscles. A muscle can consist of tens of thousands muscle fibres that are controlled by approximately 100–400 axons, depending on the size and the type of muscle.

Each motor neuron in the ventral horn of the spinal cord grey matter and the motor nuclei of cranial nerves in the brainstem is connected to multiple muscle fibres via motor end plates. The British neurophysiologist Charles Sherrington used the term motor unit (MU) to describe the relationship between a motor neuron and the skeletal muscle fibres innervated by the neuron's axon terminals. When an action potential originating from a motor neuron reaches the end-plates, neurotransmitters are released and the information is transferred electrochemically over the neuromuscular junctions to the fibres. This causes a local depolarisation of the muscle fibres. The depolarisation propagates into both directions of the fibres in the form of a so-called motor unit action potential (MUAP) causing its contraction. The number of muscle fibres per motor unit falls in is in the range of several hundreds. There are two mechanisms by which muscle force can be regulated. First, the firing rate of each activated motor unit can be increased to increase the force. Second, the number of active motor units can be increased.

In the case of an amputation, the lost limb remains represented in the brain and can be controlled by the affected person in the same way an intact limb is actuated. If the person actuates their so-called phantom limb, motor commands are transferred the same way as in able-bodied individuals and the residual muscles in the stump contract. These contractions generate EMG signals similar as in able-bodied persons, which can be picked up with surface electrodes to control the prosthesis.

1.3 EMG signal processing

The typical processing of the EMG signals for prosthesis control can include the following steps:

Filtering: To improve the signal-to-noise ratio of the raw EMG, temporal filters are commonly applied. Typically, a high-pass filter with cut-of frequency of 20–30 Hz is applied to remove any DC offset and potential motion artefacts. A low-pass filter with cut-off frequency of 300–500 Hz is applied to remove high frequency noise above the EMG spectrum, and a notch filter with 50 or 60 Hz is used to remove powerline interference.

Envelope extraction: The amplitude of the EMG increases monotonically with increasing muscle force. Therefore, it contains the most important "for the extraction" control information. Technically, this can be done by rectification and low-pass filtering, as done in conventional active electrode modules.

Windowing – feature extraction: In advanced machine-learning-based approaches, where various features are extracted from the raw EMG, the data is processed in windows of 100–250 ms duration. To minimise the delay between motor command and prosthesis reaction, the windows are typically overlapping with an increment of 20–100 ms. A broad variety of features including simple time-domain features (mean absolute value, number of zero crossings, number of slope sign changes and wavelength), as well as time-frequency features based on short-time Fourier transformation, wavelet transformation, wavelet packet transformation and auto regressive models have been proposed. Though in offline decoding scenarios, some feature sets may perform better than others, in real-time control applications such differences seem to be negligible and it has become evident that the time-domain feature set is a sufficient input source for machine-learning algorithms. Often just a measure of amplitude such as root mean square (RMS) or mean absolute value (MAV) is applied with reasonable results.

1.4   Myoelectric control algorithms

1.4.1   Basic concepts

Currently, the most often used control type is based on two myoelectric control sites located on antagonistic muscles of the residual limb, as can be seen in Figure 1.3. The EMG activity of the extensor muscles is mapped into an opening of the hand and activity of the flexor muscles is closing the hand and the controller works based on two thresholds. Typically, a proportional control is established, i.e. current through the motor(s) is controlled proportionally to the amplitude of the EMG signal. This offers the user the voluntary control of the prosthesis velocity and the grasping force. Modern prostheses may integrate more complex control mechanisms, such as internal regulation of the grasping force or a non-linear mapping between EMG amplitude and velocity or force, but the basic concepts are very similar to the classic approach that was established already in the first products.

For users with restricted anatomical conditions who can only control one channel actively, there exist also single-site control techniques. The function (open vs. close) is selected via the level (amplitude threshold) or the rate (slope threshold), or an alternation of the functions is established [6].

For children under 3 years of age, a single-side one-level voluntary opening strategy has been established. In this concept, also known as 'cookie crusher', signals above a certain threshold cause opening of the hand, and in all other cases, the hand is automatically closed.

1.4.2   Classical extensions to multiple degrees of freedom

With the classical two-channel control scheme, it is possible to control only one degree of freedom (DoF) at a time. Directly extending this concept to more DoFs by increasing the number of electrodes is usually not possible, as most users would not provide enough independent controllable EMG signals. An exception is for patients who have undergone a targeted muscle re-innervation (TMR) surgery. For other patients, heuristic approaches have been introduced to control more than one DoFs with two EMG channels. For trans-radial patients, an active wrist rotation has been established. The two most common control techniques are co-contraction control (Figure 1.4) and slope control (Figure 1.5).

In co-contraction control, the user performs a short contraction of both muscle groups at the same time, which is detected by the controller, which then switches into rotation mode. Then the two EMG signals are used to rotate the wrist in one or the other direction in a proportional way. In order to open or close the hand, the user first needs to switch back into grasping mode by performing another co-contraction. In slope control, both functions are directly accessible and the function (grasping or rotation) is selected based on the slope with which the EMG signals are raising. Slowly increasing amplitudes cause an opening or closing of the hand (depending on which channel is activated) and quickly increasing amplitudes are mapped into a supination or pronation of the prosthetic hand.

Co-contraction control

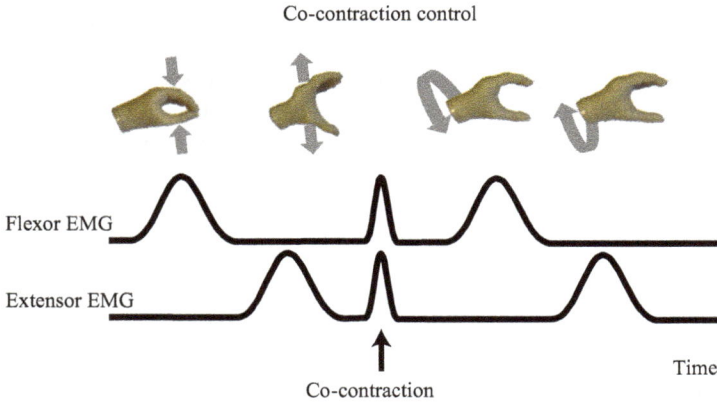

Flexor EMG

Extensor EMG

Co-contraction

Time

Figure 1.4   Co-contraction control

Slope control

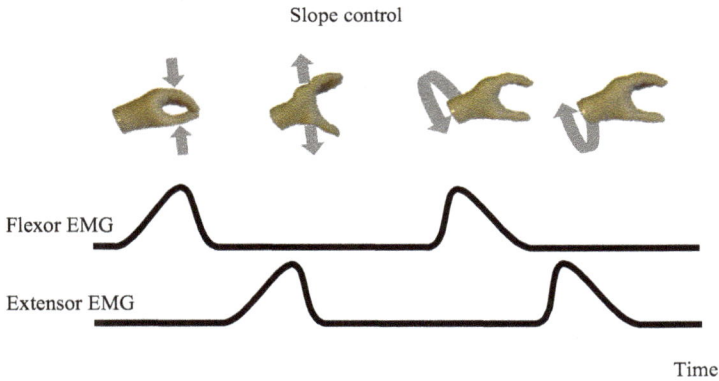

Flexor EMG

Extensor EMG

Time

Figure 1.5   Slope control

With slope control, the user can be faster than with co-contraction control, as the mode switching is omitted, but users report unintended rotations in cases they are in a rush or when they conduct reflexive motions, e.g. when they are scared. People with trans-humeral limb difference or shoulder disarticulation can use active elbow prosthesis up to three functions. Control is typically with two EMG channels, placed on the residual biceps/triceps or on deltoid/pectoralis major muscles. Typically, the user would cycle through three modes (elbow, wrist and hand) with co-contractions, which is relatively slow and cumbersome.

1.4.3 Targeted muscle re-innervation

Upon a proximal amputation more joints should be replaced but the challenge is that fewer control sites are available. A surgical approach to overcome this paradox is TMR. In this procedure, which has been introduced by Kuiken [7], the nerves of the amputated arm are surgically re-connected to more proximal, yet existing muscles that are not used anymore due to the amputation.

After shoulder disarticulation, the three major motor nerves of the arm, namely the radial, the ulnar and median nerve, are typically connected to different sections of pectoralis major muscle, the pectoralis minor muscle, serratus anterior muscle and latissimus dorsi [8].

After successful re-innervation, these breast and chest muscles contract when the person actuates his phantom limb and generates EMG signals that can be used to control a prosthesis. The re-innervated muscles can be therefore seen as natural amplifiers that transform the weak and difficult accessible neural signals of the arm nerves into stronger EMG signals that are accessible with surface electrodes. Moreover, as the muscles are spatially well separated, in the best case, up to six independent control signals are generated, which can be directly used to control three DoFs proportionally and simultaneously. For each DoF, two signals would be used in this case. In case less than six signals are available, one DoF can be controlled with one of the single-channel approaches or two DoFs with two electrodes as described earlier.

A very important, and in many cases, crucial argument for the surgery is the successful treatment of phantom limb pain and neuroma-related pain due to TMR [9].

1.4.4   Other control approaches using two EMG channels

Several commercially available prostheses offer individually actuated fingers [10]. Often the thumb is even equipped with two active DoFs. Controlling five to seven DoFs with mode switching techniques as described earlier would be inefficient. Therefore, the manufactures have predefined grasp types and offer different strategies for grasp selection. In the Bebionic hand, the thumb can be re-positioned passively with the intact hand, and for each thumb position, the user can switch between two grasp types with a button located on the dorsal side of the prosthesis. The stored grasp patterns can be configured using a smartphone app, a feature which is available for most multi-articulating prostheses. The hands of the i-Limb™ series offer a grasp selection via inertial-detected movements of the prosthesis in one out of four directions, after the user initiates the function with an EMG trigger. Also here the grasps can be configured via a smartphone app. Another concept is to select the grasp type with radio-frequency identification (RFID) tags read by the prosthesis that are placed on various objects or in different rooms.

Figure 1.6 depicts our interpretation of the prosthesis control space. In this section, we aim to describe this control space and set the scene for introducing advanced prosthesis control methods. In this figure, on the horizontal axis, we have 'estimation of the user intent' and on the vertical axis, we have 'user adaptation'. With these two axes, we aim to contrast the two methods of machine learning and human learning for prosthesis control, benchmarking them again the standard thresholding approach.

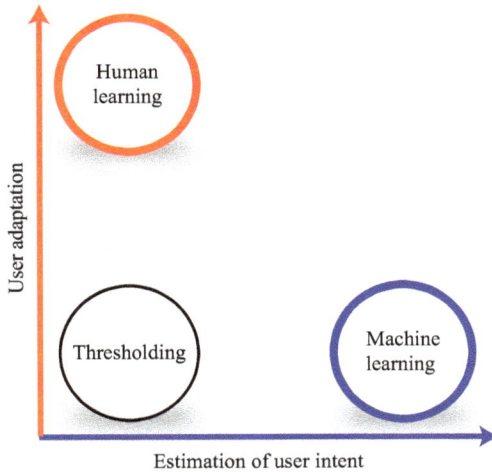

Figure 1.6   The prosthesis control space

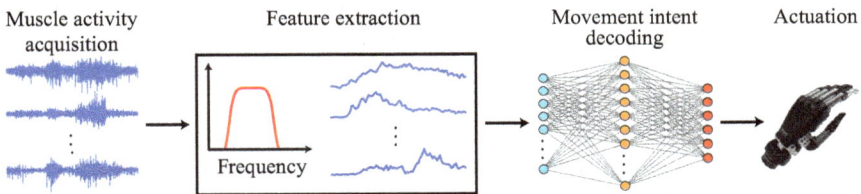

Figure 1.7   Machine learning for prosthesis control

1.4.5   Machine learning

To overcome the limitations of the classical myoelectric control approaches, significant research has been conducted to employ machine-learning techniques to extract a higher number of control signals from the residual muscles starting in the 1970s [11].

Machine learning for the control of a prosthesis aims to decode user intentions or motor commands such that an intended movement maps to its prosthetic substitute. Figure 1.7 depicts this approach. When using EMG, inertial or other input signals, the detected movement or grasp intentions are usually limited to commonly used ones [12,13]. During calibration, the machine-learning algorithm requires training data representative of each grasp to train a classifier, which then categorises new samples during actual use.

The classification approach (Figure 1.7) offers significant improvement of the intuitiveness and ease of use of the prosthetic device when compared to the thresholding approach. However, there are two key challenges or limitations. First is that

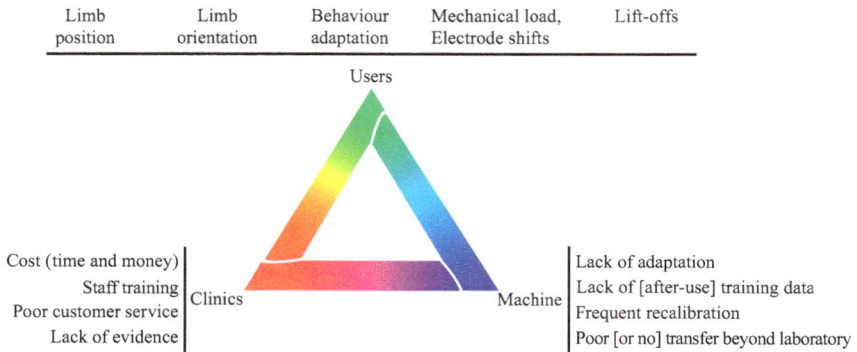

Figure 1.8   Myriad of challenges in using pure machine learning for prosthetic control

classification still underactuates the prosthesis and that remarkably limits the functionality and the versatility of the device. This is because the user can utilise only a small set of pre-determined grips, despite that the device itself offers the possibility of controlling each DoF, typically six, individually. The second challenge is that classification inevitably is sequential in nature, that is, only one grip or movement can be active at any time, as opposed to the smooth, continuous and asynchronous finger movement exhibited by the natural hand.

Researchers have been working towards the continuous and simultaneous control of multiple DoFs to radically improve the dexterity of prosthetic hands [14]. The main objective of continuous control has been to restore wrist function [15–18]. However, recently many have tried to address the challenge of reconstructing the kinematics (position or velocity) of prosthetic digits offline [19–24] and in real time [24–27].

Published literature suggests that when a machine learning-based controller is trained for the desired outputs, it could provide a viable method of prosthesis control [28]. Specifically, pattern recognition of the EMG signals has reached the market [29,30]. The core challenges that limit the robustness of this control approach in terms of ensuring training data adequately characterises real-world data [31]. Figure 1.8 lists some of the other challenges associated with machine-learning-based approaches that researchers try to address currently.

1.4.6   Human learning

Recently, human learning-based methods have been introduced in experimental settings [32–39]. It is promised that they offer an alternative paradigm to machine learning-based methods for controlling prosthetic hands. These methods rely upon closed-loop feedback, typically visual, to help the users adapt their muscle behaviour. Importantly, within this paradigm, the patterns of muscular activity used for control can differ from those that control biological limbs, but with practice, users can learn these new functional patterns of muscular activity and use them for control. It is envisaged that these methods can result in enhanced control without increasing device complexity. More recently, insight into the clinical readiness of human learning-based approach has been provided in [40]. Although early results indicate potential success, there is still a long route before the human learning methods could be used in the clinic.

References

[1] Farina D, Jiang N, Rehbaum H, *et al.* The extraction of neural information from the surface EMG for the control of upper-limb prostheses: emerging avenues and challenges. IEEE Transactions on Neural Systems and Rehabilitation Engineering. 2014;22(4):797–809.

[2] OrthoTeam. Body-powered prosthesis [Website]. OrthoTeam; 2020 [cited 2020-06-06]. Available from: https://produkte.ortho-team.ch/de-de/Category/ Index / p - OA - Prothese - Eigenkraft?path = Produktewelt%2Fprothesen%2Fh-prothesen-armprothesen%2Fg-armprothesen-oberarmprothesen.

[3] Reiter R. Eine neue Elektrokunsthand. Grenzgebiete der Medizin. 1948; 1(4):133–135.

[4] Sherman ED. A Russian bioelectric-controlled prosthesis. Canadian Medical Association Journal. 1964;91(24):1268–1270.

[5] Purves D. Neuroscience. Cary, NC, USA: Oxford University Press; 2012.

[6] Muzumdar A. Powered upper limb prostheses: control, implementation and clinical application. Berlin Heidelberg: Springer; 2004.

[7] Kuiken TA, Li G, Lock BA, *et al.* Targeted muscle reinnervation for real-time myoelectric control of multifunction artificial arms. JAMA. 2009;301(6): 619–628.

[8] Miller LA, Stubblefield KA, Lipschutz RD, Lock BA, and Kuiken TA. Improved myoelectric prosthesis control using targeted reinnervation surgery: a case series. IEEE Transactions on Neural Systems and Rehabilitation Engineering. 2008;16(1):46–50.

[9] Dumanian GA, Potter BK, Mioton LM, *et al.* Targeted muscle reinnervation treats neuroma and phantom pain in major limb amputees: a randomized clinical trial. Annals of surgery. 2019;270(2):238–246.

[10] Belter JT, Segil JL, Dollar AM, and Weir RF. Mechanical design and performance specifications of anthropomorphic prosthetic hands: a review. Journal of Rehabilitation Research and Development. 2013;50(5):599–618.

[11] Graupe D and Cline WK. Functional separation of EMG signals via ARMA identification methods for prosthesis control purposes. IEEE Transactions on Systems, Man and Cybernetics. 1975;SMC-5(2):252–259.

[12] Hudgins B, Parker P, and Scott RN. A new strategy for multifunction myoelectric control. IEEE Transactions on Biomedical Engineering. 1993;40(1):82–94.

[13] Englehart K and Hudgins B. A robust, real-time control scheme for multifunction myoelectric control. IEEE Transactions on Biomedical Engineering. 2003;50(7):848–854.

[14]   Fougner A, Stavdahl Ø, Kyberd PJ, Losier YG, and Parker PA. Control of upper limb prostheses: terminology and proportional myoelectric control—a review. IEEE Transactions on Neural Systems and Rehabilitation Engineering. 2012;20(5):663–677.

[15]   Muceli S, Jiang N, and Farina D. Extracting signals robust to electrode number and shift for online simultaneous and proportional myoelectric control by factorization algorithms. IEEE Transactions on Neural Systems and Rehabilitation Engineering. 2014;22(3):623–633.

[16]   Hahne JM, Schweisfurth MA, Koppe M, and Farina D. Simultaneous control of multiple functions of bionic hand prostheses: performance and robustness in end users. Science Robotics. 2018;3(19):eaat3630.

[17]   Jiang N, Vujaklija I, Rehbaum H, Graimann B, and Farina D. Is accurate mapping of EMG signals on kinematics needed for precise online myoelectric control? IEEE Transactions on Neural Systems and Rehabilitation Engineering. 2014;22(3):549–558.

[18]   Smith LH, Kuiken TA, and Hargrove LJ. Real-time simultaneous and proportional myoelectric control using intramuscular EMG. Journal of Neural Engineering. 2014;11(6):066013.

[19]   Afshar P and Matsuoka Y. Neural-based control of a robotic hand: evidence for distinct muscle strategies. In: Proc. IEEE Int. Conf. Robot. Autom. (ICRA); vol. 5; 2004. pp. 4633–4638.

[20]   Smith RJ, Tenore F, Huberdeau D, Etienne-Cummings R, and Thakor NV. Continuous decoding of finger position from surface EMG signals for the control of powered prostheses. In: Proc. IEEE Int. Conf. Eng. Med. Biol. Soc. (EMBC); 2008. p. 197–200.

[21]   Ngeo JG, Tamei T, and Shibata T. Continuous and simultaneous estimation of finger kinematics using inputs from an EMG-to-muscle activation model. Journal of NeuroEngineering and Rehabilitation. 2014;11(1):122.

[22]   Krasoulis A, Vijayakumar S, and Nazarpour K. Evaluation of regression methods for the continuous decoding of finger movement from surface EMG and accelerometry. In: Proc. IEEE/EMBS Int. Conf. Neural Eng. (NER); 2015. pp. 631–634.

[23]   Xiloyannis M, Gavriel C, Thomik AAC, and Faisal AA. Gaussian process autoregression for simultaneous proportional multi-modal prosthetic control with natural hand kinematics. IEEE Transactions on Neural Systems and Rehabilitation Engineering. 2017;25(10):1785–1801.

[24]   Krasoulis A and Nazarpour K. Myoelectric digit action decoding with multi-label, multi-class classification: an offline analysis. bioRxiv. 2020. Available from: https://www.biorxiv.org/content/early/2020/03/25/2020.03.24.005710.

[25]   Krasoulis A, Kyranou I, Erden M, Nazarpour K, and Vijayakumar S. Improved prosthetic hand control with concurrent use of myoelectric and inertial measurements. Journal of NeuroEngineering and Rehabilitation. 2017;14:71.

[26]   Smith RJ, Huberdeau D, Tenore F, and Thakor NV. Real-time myoelectric decoding of individual finger movements for a virtual target task. In: Proc. IEEE Int. Conf. Eng. Med. Biol. Soc. (EMBC); 2009. p. 2376–2379.

[27] Ngeo JG, Tamei T, Shibata T, *et al*. Control of an optimal finger exoskeleton based on continuous joint angle estimation from EMG signals. In: Proc. IEEE Int. Conf. Eng. Med. Biol. Soc. (EMBC); 2013. p. 338–341.

[28] Ortiz-Catalan M, Håkansson B, and Brånemark R. Real-time and simultaneous control of artificial limbs based on pattern recognition algorithms. IEEE Transactions on Neural Systems and Rehabilitation Engineering. 2014;22(4): 756–764.

[29] Coapt L. Coapt engineering; 2019. [Online; accessed 27-August-2019]. https://coaptengineering.com.

[30] Ottobock G. Myo plus pattern recognition; 2019. [Online; accessed 27-August-2019]. https://www.ottobock.co.uk/prosthetics/upper-limb-prosthetics/product-systems/myo-plus/.

[31] Scheme EJ and Englehart KB. Electromyogram pattern recognition for control of powered upper-limb prostheses: State of the art and challenges for clinical use. Journal of Rehabilitation Research and Development. 2011;48(6): 643–660.

[32] Radhakrishnan SM, Baker SN, and Jackson A. Learning a novel myoelectric-controlled interface task. Journal of Neurophysiology. 2008;100(4): 2397–2408.

[33] Pistohl T, Cipriani C, Jackson A, and Nazarpour K. Abstract and proportional myoelectric control for multi-fingered hand prostheses. Annals of Biomedical Engineering. 2013;41(12):2687–2698.

[34] Antuvan CW, Ison M, and Artemiadis P. Embedded human control of robots using myoelectric interfaces. IEEE Transactions on Neural Systems and Rehabilitation Engineering. 2014;22(4):820–827.

[35] Ison M and Artemiadis P. Proportional myoelectric control of robots: muscle synergy development drives performance enhancement, retainment, and generalization. IEEE Transactions on Robotics. 2015;31(2):259–268.

[36] Pistohl T, Josh D, Ganesh G, Jackson A, and Nazarpour K. Artificial proprioceptive feedback for myoelectric control. IEEE Transactions on Neural Systems Rehabilitation Engineering. 2015;23(3):498–507.

[37] Segil JL and Weir RF. Novel postural control algorithm for control of multifunctional myoelectric prosthetic hands. Journal of Rehabilitation Research and Development. 2015;52(4):449–466.

[38] Dyson M, Barnes J, and Nazarpour K. Myoelectric control with abstract decoders. Journal of Neural Engineering. 2018;15(5):056003.

[39] Dyson M, Dupan S, Jones H, and Nazarpour K. Learning, generalisation, scalability of abstract myoelectric control. IEEE Transactions on Neural Systems and Rehabilitation Engineering. 2020;28(7):1539–1547.

[40] Segil JL, Kaliki R, Uellendahl J, and Weir RF. A myoelectric postural control algorithm for persons with transradial amputation: a consideration of clinical readiness. IEEE Robotics and Automation Magazine. 2020;27(1):77–86.

Chapter 2
Methods to design bespoke sockets
Sarah Day[1]

The socket is an integral and important part of the prosthetic limb, providing link between body and technology. The quality of this connection must be considered as we strive towards embodiment of the prosthetic limb. The purpose of the socket is not just to provide a container for the residual limb but to provide a vessel where biomechanical forces can be transmitted from the body to the prosthetic componentry in the most energy-efficient manner while protecting the underlying tissues. The residual limb consists of bone surrounded by an envelope of soft tissues, including muscles which may no longer have insertion points. As the bone is able to move within the envelope of soft tissues, poor transmission of force and discomfort within the prosthesis can occur. Stabilising tissues to minimise bone movement within the socket is considered one of the primary goals in designing and constructing a well-fitting socket.

2.1 What makes a good socket?

It is difficult to define what makes a good socket. Factors such as comfort are often used to determine the success of a socket. This subjective measure, however, is difficult to quantify and a person's perception of comfort can change day-to-day according to how the wearer is feeling or what tasks are being performed. In addition to comfort, prosthetists consider factors such as the volume of the socket, preserving the range of motion of intact joints and the quality of suspension when determining if the fit and design of the socket is appropriate. The final judgement, however, always belongs to the wearer as a prosthetic limb must be comfortable and useful if it is to used regularly. While it is difficult to quantify what makes a good socket, we do know that prosthetic limb wearers are less likely to use a prosthesis with an ill-fitting socket. Socket discomfort is frequently reported as a compounding factor for prosthesis rejection. Other socket-related factors which contribute to limb abandonment include weight, heat, difficulty donning and poor suspension [1–5].

Every person who wears a prosthetic arm is unique, and therefore the prosthetic socket must be custom-made to meet the individual requirements of the wearer. Design criteria will be established following an assessment of the wearer's anatomy, needs and preferences.

[1]National Centre for Prosthetics and Orthotics, Department of Biomedical Engineering, University of Strathclyde, Glasgow, UK

The health and condition of the residual limb depends greatly on the surgery that was performed and on the person's recovery. Poor surgical technique or post-amputation complications can result in socket-fitting issues later. Ideally the amputation should result in a mid-length residual limb (1/3 to 1/2 of the original bone length). A mid-length residual limb is preferable when limb-fitting as the limb will have a long enough lever arm and muscle strength to allow good powerful movement within a prosthesis while having space for prosthetic componentry to be fitted without affecting overall limb length. Maintaining overall limb length is important for cosmesis, body symmetry and proprioception. Complications that may occur following amputation surgery include bony spurs, nerve pain, muscle imbalance and loose tissue. These would be identified during the patient assessment process conducted by the prosthetist and must be considered when designing an appropriate socket.

2.2   Socket design considerations

The prosthetic socket is a custom-made product and should be designed by a competent person, namely a prosthetist, following a medical history and assessment of the user. The exact design of the socket will be influenced by factors such as skin quality, scarring, what the prosthesis will be used for, and how it will be powered.

Factors influencing the socket design

When designing a socket, there are a number of key features that must be considered. These features cannot be considered individually as each feature will influence the others:

- the tightness of the socket (socket fit);
- stability within the socket;
- how the socket will be held on (suspension);
- how high the socket will extend on the arm (trimlines);
- how easy the socket will be to don/doff; and
- what materials the socket will be made of.

In the following sub-sections, we review these factors.

2.2.1   Socket fit

When we discuss socket biomechanics, stiffest path principle and energy efficiency, we normally assume that the resultant socket will be tight-fitting. However, the human body is subject to volume changes and these will affect the tightness of the prosthetic socket on the residual limb. While volume fluctuations are not as troublous in the upper limbs as in the lower limbs, prosthetic limb wearers will notice variations in socket fit between morning and evening, from day to day and over time. Traditionally, wearers of cosmetic and body-powered prostheses have used stump socks to manage any changes in volume. Stump socks are tubular-shaped socks similar to those worn on the feet. They are available in various lengths and thicknesses, and users will often wear socks in layers, adding and removing them to accommodate volume fluctuations. In addition to reducing the biomechanical efficiency of the socket by introducing compressible layers, the practice of using multiple socks under the socket can increase skin temperature and bulkiness. Socket volume cannot be managed in this way within a myoelectric prosthesis, as the electrodes need to be in direct contact with the skin. There is a growing trend for sockets with adjustable volume. These designs often incorporate a clamshell construction with a dial adjustable lacing system, such as a Boa device. Advantages of such systems are that small changes in volume can be accommodated, and donning and doffing the socket is easier; however, the socket will be bulkier and care must be taken to ensure that the shape matching aspects of the socket, and electrode positions, are not compromised.

2.2.2 Stability

The socket provides the physical and mechanical link between the body and the prosthetic componentry. During limb movement, the remaining bone will move within its envelope of soft tissue. In order to transmit forces effectively, it is essential that the soft tissues of the residual limb are stabilised as this will minimise unwanted bone and tissue movement. Internal shear forces caused by longitudinal displacement or transverse and rotational displacement of tissues are known to cause damage to tissue. To minimise internal shear forces, it is important that the socket environment provides a stiff coupling between the bone and the tissues. This will help one to ensure that there is minimal pistoning both within the tissues of the limb, and between the socket and the skin. Vulnerable areas of the residual limb, such as the tissues around the scar or those stretched over the cut end of bone, are less likely to breakdown in sockets which adhere to the stiff coupling principle [6]. Pistoning between the socket and skin is exasperated by the inclusion of heavy componentry within the limb build. Reducing pistoning must be a priority when designing a socket and can be managed by incorporating a suitable suspension system. Soft tissues are at higher risk of breakdown if they are subjected to high pressures applied over a prolonged period. Studies have shown that pressures should not exceed 15–20 mmHg for extended periods [7]. While pressures inside a prosthetic socket often exceed this level, the risk is minimised by wearing time. This is well documented in lower limb prosthetic sockets, where pressure is off-loaded by the cyclic loading during the gait cycle [7,8] but remains an underexplored area within upper limb prosthetic design. Reducing shear pressure is critical for preventing deep tissue injury [9,10]. One method which prosthetists use to reduce socket pressures is to apply the principle of total contact socket design. In essence, this is where forces are spread over as large a surface area as possible based on the formula pressure = force/area. Surface matching is critical in avoiding high pressures over bony prominences and associated boundary pressure gradients.

Contouring the socket, through either surface matching to the underlying bony anatomy or compressing soft tissues, will help one to prevent rotation of the socket and subsequent skin damage caused by torsional forces. Rotation of sockets is commonly an issue when trimlines are kept low, for example, in transradial sockets which do not extend over the elbow and in under-the-shoulder trans-humeral designs.

A number of socket designs, exist which do not adhere to the total contact principles of socket design. Instead, these have struts which make contact with the arm, providing stability for the prosthesis. Examples of these include the WILMER, socket-less socket and high-fidelity (Hi-Fi) socket.

2.2.3 Suspension

A good socket should not piston on the arm while being worn. During lifting, the additional weight of the object being carried may cause the prosthetic arm to slip distally. In addition, during flexion and extension of the arm, a prosthetic socket that is not adequately anchored can move on the soft tissues causing friction and potential skin breakdown. To avoid slippage, it is essential that the socket is securely suspended on to the arm. Unless an osseointegration procedure has been performed, most sockets will utilise either skin traction, an indirect skeletal suspension method, or harnessing to suspend the prosthesis to the body. Harnessing is the method of attaching the prosthesis to the body using straps. Normally two or more straps will be attached to the socket, and then the strapping will run up the arm, across the back and under the axilla of the other arm. Buckles or Velcro may be included to allow the wearer some adjustability for bulky or light-weight clothing. While harnessing can be used for proximal levels of amputation, it is rarely used with below elbow prostheses as the straps can be cumbersome for the wearer. In addition, the harnessing process is time consuming, strapping stretches over time, and is difficult to keep clean. Issues with harnessing are reported as reasons for limb abandonment.

Indirect skeletal suspension is where the socket or an accessory is shaped to resist slippage. Shaping the socket so that it is narrow above a bony prominence will provide a resistance to downwards slippage. There are many methods of indirect skeletal suspension that can be used, while some rely solely on surface matching of the underlying bony anatomy, other methods apply forces to soft tissue above the bony prominence to enhance the effect. This technique can be incorporated within the design of the socket itself, such as in a supracondylar or supra-olecranon-styled socket, or provided within an accessory such as a humeral cuff. To enable easy donning of the socket, trimlines, and material construction will need to be considered. Cuff suspension, a form of indirect skeletal suspension, where the prosthesis is suspended by an adjustable circumferential force proximal to the socket, used to be a common prescription. It is no longer frequently used in clinical prosthetic designs but features within many open-source socket designs within the additive manufacture community. In disarticulations, indirect skeletal suspension can often be achieved through surface matching around the distal condyles. This is beneficial as it means that the socket does not need to extend to the proximal joint but leads to issues donning and doffing the socket.

Fleshy residual limbs can be suspended using skin traction, with or without a suction valve or vacuum. These sockets are normally very tight and the wearer may need to use a sleeve to pull their tissues into the socket. Additional shaping can be applied around the proximal trimline to mould the socket over the anatomy to provide additional indirect skeletal suspension.

As with lower limb prosthetic sockets, a silicone or gel suspension liner can be used as the suspension component. The liner has a high coefficient of friction which means that it sticks firmly to the skin unless it is rolled off. The liner is rolled onto the skin then the socket is donned over the top. The socket will connect to the liner by either a lanyard, pin and lock system or a vacuum. Liners provide a secure method of suspension providing that an appropriate sized liner has been selected. A limited size range of liners is available from commercial suppliers but they also can be custom-made in prosthetic workshops by laminating silicone over a mould of the residual limb. Trans-humeral prosthetic sockets are normally suspended using either harnessing, vacuum suspension or a roll-on liner with lock/lanyard.

2.2.4 Trimlines

Maintaining range of motion of intact anatomical joints is a key aim in prosthetic design as any restriction in movement could lead to soft tissue contractures and/or compensatory body movements. Keeping the trimlines of the socket low will ensure that the range of motion at proximal joints is not limited. It is not always possible, however, to keep trimlines low as objectives such as maximising surface area or providing indirect skeletal suspension often mean that a compromise needs to be made. For example, the trimlines on a short transradial socket will normally extend above the cubital fold. This will block the amount of elbow flexion possible, and unless an element of pre-flexion has been incorporated into the alignment, the prosthetic user may be required to adopt compensatory movements in order to complete their activities of daily living. Full elbow extension will be restricted in most sockets which extend over the olecranon such as the supra-olecranon, Brim and Muenster sockets. Range of motion, along with other socket characteristics are easily checked when a transparent diagnostic socket is fitted prior to fabricating the definitive socket. Figure 2.1 illustrates how elbow flexion and extension can be limited by the trimlines, and also how contact between the arm and posterior socket is lost during elbow extension.

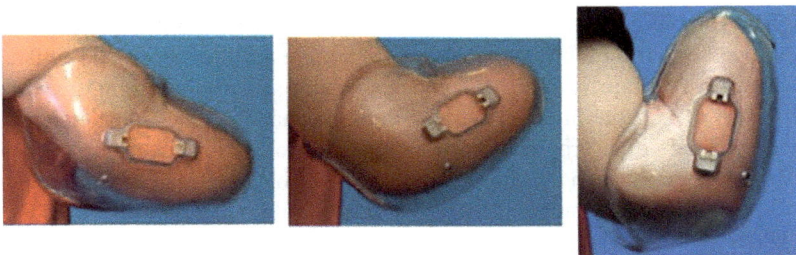

Figure 2.1   A diagnostic socket being used to test socket fit, range of motion and ease of donning

It is common, especially in bilateral amputees, to remove socket material around the elbow itself. This must be accounted for prior to manufacturing the socket as cutting away material can weaken the structure of the socket. Leaving the elbow open can enhance sensation for some prosthesis wearers; for example, they will be able to feel clothing through the socket. As illustrated in Figure 2.1, the posterior socket loses contact with the arm during elbow extension, and a relief is normally required for the olecranon at full flexion, therefore there are few disadvantages to removing this section of the socket. Wearers also report that their arm will be cooler if the socket has an open elbow. The challenges associated with determining the optimal trimline height will vary according to the physical presentation of the wearer and the design of socket being made. Trimline height is often finalised at the time of delivery of the prosthesis and can often be altered later.

2.2.5   Donning and doffing the prosthesis

In addition to maintaining the range of motion of remaining joints, the trimlines of the socket will influence how easily the prosthesis can be donned and doffed. It is important that a person with limb absence should be able to don and doff their prostheses independently. This means that the process should be simple and straightforward as it will need to be conducted one handed, or by using residual limbs, other body segments or assistive devices if the wearer has an upper limb bilateral absence. In practice, sockets with lower trimlines will be easier to don/doff. The addition of a liner which needs to be rolled on and off, a pull-in sleeve, valve, straps, buckles, etc. will add complication and may be a prohibiting factor for a bilateral prosthetic user. Fitting a diagnostic socket, which is a temporary socket used by prosthetists to assess fit and suspension, can be a useful step as this will enable the wearer to practice donning and doffing the socket before the definitive is made.

2.2.6   Materials for sockets

When fabricating a socket, most builds comprise an inner socket and an outer socket. The inner socket will be formed over a modified cast or model of the residual limb and should be designed according to total contact principles. The outer socket is formed around the inner socket and connects the socket to the rest of the prosthetic limb. Channels can be built between the two sockets for cables to run through. In some cases, for example in cosmetic prosthetic limbs, the inner and outer sockets may be bonded together during fabrication to produce a more seamless cosmetic finish.

The stiffest path principle is the concept often used when designing prosthetic sockets. This means that in order to transmit biomechanics forces most efficiently, a stiff medium should be provided. For this reason, prosthetic sockets are commonly made from materials such as reinforced acrylic or polyester resin. Rigid materials, however, can restrict the range of motion and so flexible materials are often used in areas where a stiff socket is not crucial. This can be, for example, in the wings of the socket to allow easier donning of the socket and near the trimlines to enable a few extra degrees of movement while still managing soft tissue volume. As illustrated in Figure 2.2, a traditional laminated socket is fabricated over a positive mould of the residual limb. Layers of fabric such as cotton, carbon fibre, fibreglass and nylon are impregnated under vacuum with a thermosetting resin which is hardened by polymerisation. The material properties of the socket are determined by the materials used in the base lay-up, including fibre length and the direction they are orientated, and the resin matrix. By using a combination of materials within the lay-up and resins of different rigidity, it is possible to create a socket with areas of stiffness and flexibility.

Compressible materials such as foams, commonly used within lower limb prosthetic sockets, are not routinely used in upper limb prosthetics. This is in part because the loads experienced by upper limbs are not as high as in the lower limb, and also because compressible materials add bulk to the socket which reduces the cosmetic appearance. While foams are not commonly used, some wearers can benefit from a silicone liner or inner socket. A roll-on silicone liner, worn next to the skin and under the socket, can protect the residual limb from shear forces and assist in scar healing. Silicone liners used along with a lanyard and cleat, or pin and lock, can provide effective suspension of the prosthesis. Examples of commercial and custom-made silicone roll-on liners are shown in Figure 2.3. One advantage of using silicone sleeve suspension is that the trimlines of the socket can often be kept lower, as suspension is not reliant on the anatomy at the distal end of the bone proximal. Assuming that the trimlines are high enough to ensure suitable distribution of forces, the anatomical joint can be left free of socket material and therefore the range of motion at that joint will be optimised and a more cosmetic finish may be achieved. Roll-on silicone liners are available to purchase commercially, but in a small range of sizes. An alternative approach is to fabricate a custom roll-on liner by laminating silicone over a mould of the residual limb. While this adds an additional step to the fabrication process, it is a cost-effective method of incorporating a silicone liner within a prosthesis for people whose arm measurements fall out with the commercial product range.

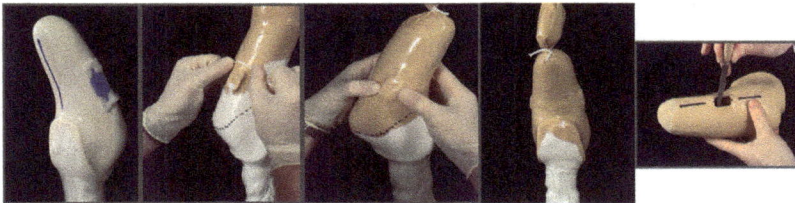

Figure 2.2   Socket lamination

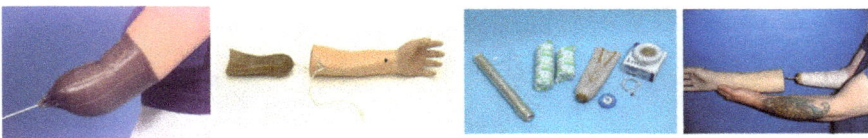

*Figure 2.3   Examples of silicone roll-on liners: custom-made laminated liner (left)
and commercial liner (right)*

Another method of combining flexibility and rigidity within the socket is to fabricate a socket with a flexible inner socket and a rigid shell. Flexible materials such as ethylene-vinyl acetate copolymers or silicone formed over a mould of the residual limb will produce an inner socket in which volume is contained while allowing flexibility at the trimlines for added comfort and the range of motion. The rigid shell provides structural support and the connection to prosthetic componentry.

Socket hygiene is essential within any prescription. When enclosing the residual limb, the temperature of the skin will be increased, and most wearers will experience an increase in perspiration. Excessive heat is a common complaint and reason for prosthesis abandonment. Bacteria can thrive within a prosthetic socket that is not regularly cleaned. Prosthetic sockets can be difficult to clean, especially if they contain electronic components, holes and channels. It is recommended that stump socks, if used, are replaced daily and washed in between wear. Sockets and silicone liners should be cleaned at the end of the day with an antibacterial wipe and left to air-dry.

Consideration must be given to the quality of the material used. It is advisable that only materials which are classed as medical grade and safe for human use should be used in areas of the socket which have contact with the skin. The European Commission and ISO Standards have produced guidance documents which classified medical devices and the materials which can be used within prosthetic sockets.

2.2.7   Shape capture

To create a bespoke socket, the measurements and shape of the person's residual limb must be captured. Prosthetists traditionally use a combination of measurements and a negative plaster cast of the limb to obtain this information. Obtaining a good a plaster cast such as that illustrated in Figure 2.4, relies on prosthetist skill, and quality and can vary. In recent years scanning has become more popular as a shape capture method. Whilst scanning has its own disadvantages, it is a repeatable procedure which is cleaner for both the prosthetist and the patient. There is a lot of variability in scanners in relation to cost, accuracy and usability. Cheap scanners, costing a few hundred pounds, can provide reasonable images with a lower degree of accuracy. For more accurate work, for example if creating a high cosmetic finish, a more accurate scanner

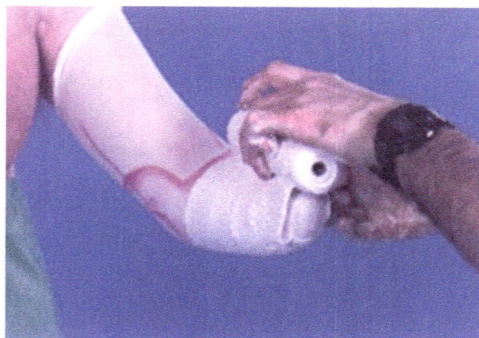

Figure 2.4   Casting a transradial arm

would be required. Tips for ensuring a good scan include adding reflective markers over anatomical landmarks. This not only assists with tracking during the scanning process itself but also helps identify the anatomical landmarks required when doing a CAD modification.

After the limb has been scanned, the file must be uploaded to a suitable CAD package. Likewise if a plaster cast has been taken, the mould should then be filled with plaster of Paris to form a positive mould of the residual limb. This positive mould can either be scanned to make a digital image for CAD or can be modified manually using traditional prosthetist plaster skills.

The process of modification of the image/positive model is critical for obtaining a well-fitting socket. In most cases, the volume of the model must be reduced to stabilise the tissues. The amount of volume reduction required will depend on the individual's features and the type of socket being made. Reliefs over bony prominences and cut end of bones are commonly built in to the socket design. During the modification process, the trimlines of the socket should be finalised. The trimlines should be set at a height that maximises surface area, thus minimising socket forces, but allows minimal interference with the range of movement and enables the socket to be donned easily. Longer residual limbs will often require lower trimlines, particularly if the socket extends over the proximal joint. A short residual limb may require very high trimlines, to prevent the residual limb from popping out of the socket during flexion.

2.3   Electrode placement

Myoelectrodes are commonly used as a switch within myoelectric prostheses. In myo control, the electrode detects changes in the electrical activity on the skin surface caused by calcium being released prior to a muscle contraction. The electrode is normally positioned wherever the signal is strongest, normally over the muscle belly, but its position may need to be moved to avoid scar tissue or trimlines/cut outs within the socket. Care must be taken to ensure that the electrode remains fully in contact with the skin throughout the entire range of motion. Electrode placement should be determined at the time of assessment, when the socket is being planned. It is not appropriate to determine this when the wearer is not present.

2.4   Task-specific devices

Success of a prosthetic limb should not be based on wearing time. When and where a person with limb absence chooses to use a prosthetic limb will vary according to the activities they are carrying out, the social environment and their limb health. It is widely acknowledged that by wearing a prosthetic socket, users will experience lower levels of touch feedback than if they were to use their residual limb to conduct a task. This along with the ability to grasp objects in the elbow crease is sufficient reason that many, especially congenital absence, choose either not to wear a prosthesis or to wear one only at selective times.

For a prosthesis to be successful, it must be comfortable and serve a useful purpose. That purpose may be functional or cosmetic, and it may be required daily, or less frequently. Useful might mean that it helps the wearer to perform a task, or it might fulfil a cosmetic or physiological need. Day and Wands-Silva [11] found that children with congenital BE absence who have a prosthetic or assistive device are most likely to use it for bimanual tasks or for leisure activities such as sports or music. For this reason, a prosthetic limb, or assistive device, could be considered as a task-specific tool. Task-specific tools have commonly been used with traditional body-powered prostheses fitted with a wrist unit that allows the terminal device to be interchanged. This makes the prosthesis multifunctional. At times, the user may choose to have a hand-shaped terminal device, other times, for example when fine grasp is required he/she may select a split hook, or a passive device can be fitted such as a gripper to secure vegetables during peeling or a typing appliance. The versatility of having interchangeable terminal devices is beneficial; however, it is costly to provide multiple terminal devices and can be inconvenient and sometimes awkward for the user to physically change these.

Rather than designing a multifunctional device, it is often more effective to design task-specific prostheses or devices. This is an area of prosthetic design that involves creativity and problem solving, and any device must be designed in consultation with the wearer to ensure a successful outcome. Non-conventional designs will require risk assessment to be performed before delivery of the device. Children are commonly provided with cycling devices which allow them to bimanually hold the handlebars of a bicycle or a scooter. Brakes are normally rerouted to be operated by the sound side. A feature of this device is that the user must be able to detach themselves from the bike quickly. This is important to prevent serious injury if the child were to fall off the bike, as it may be dangerous for them to physically be attached to the bike. This can be done either by designing a device that can be detached quickly from the handlebars or by the user pulling themselves free from the device. Another area where children will commonly use a device is when learning a musical instrument. Music is known to have therapeutic benefits and is included in the national curriculum. Exclusion from such activities would be detrimental to the child. Musical devices are normally designed on a bespoke case. A simple socket or band is usually made with an attachment to either hold, support or operate the instrument. Devices like these are likely to be worn every week during lessons but may be abandoned once the child has moved on to a new hobby. For this reason, a low-cost built may be appropriate, but as with all assistive devices, quality must not be compromised as this could affect the child's ability to progress. The strength and durability of the device must be considered as a prosthesis or assistive device that breaks is not useful and may prevent the child from participating in tasks. There are many open source 3D printed patterns available on the internet. Some of these might be suitable for task-specific activities, but the fit, appropriateness and strength of the device should be considered before it is provided.

2.5   Common transradial socket designs

Transradial prostheses are the most commonly prescribed upper limb prosthetic devices [12]. There are many socket designs suitable for residual limbs at this level, and selection of the type to be used will be determined following a full patient assessment. Images of selected socket designs are shown in Figure 2.6. When fitting a short fleshy residual limb, the socket must encompass a large section of the arm, commonly extending to the elbow crease or beyond, to maximise surface area. Many people who have short fleshy residual limbs will have underdeveloped skeletal anatomy, and length discrepancies may be present if the limb was absent at birth or amputated in childhood. Sockets for this level can be designed to worn either directly next to the skin, or with an interface liner or sock.

The Muenster socket was created by Hepp and Kuhn in the 1950s for persons with short residual limbs and is instantly recognisable due to a convexity on the anterior trim. This is a tight-fitting self-suspending socket with high trimlines to enclose all tissues below the elbow. An anterior–posterior compression force is applied to the triceps tendon and either side of the biceps tendon. This creates a relief for the biceps tendon and the Muenster socket iconic appearance. The socket has high trimlines and as a result both flexion and extension of the elbow will be limited. Prosthetists commonly compensate for this reduction in elbow flexion by pre-flexing the alignment of components to ensure that the prosthesis remains functional for body-centred activities. The Brim socket is a tight-fitting socket that relies on skin traction for suspension. Additional suspension is provided by a circumferential shallow grove which is cut into the plaster model at the level above the humeral condyles during cast modification. This grove provides minimal indirect skeletal suspension in people with underdeveloped condyles, but when incorporated within a tight-fitting socket it increases the skin traction. Like other sockets designed for short fleshy residual limbs, the Brim socket restricts elbow flexion and extension due to its high trimlines (Figure 2.5). Anatomically contoured interface (TRAC) is an aggressively modified hybrid of the Muenster and Northwestern sockets. This design requires a flexible inner socket. The socket is contoured in five areas to stabilise muscle groups and prevent rotation of the socket.

When considering a socket design for a mid-length residual limb, there are many tried and tested socket designs to choose from. Selection will normally be determined by suspension type and prosthetist preference. In these designs, the trimlines are lower anteriorly, allowing more normal elbow flexion. The Northwestern socket is perhaps the most famous transradial socket design. Created by John Billock at Northwestern University in the 1970s, this socket utilises a tight medio-lateral diameter fit over the humeral epicondyles for suspension. This is accompanied by a low anterior trimline, extending up to 45% of the overall length of the socket. Due to the tight M/L dimension of the design, a progressive wear program may be required to build up tolerance to pressure above the condyles.

A successor of the Northwestern socket is the Strathclyde Supra Olecranon Socket (SSOS) designed by Bill Dykes at the University of Strathclyde in the 1980s. The aim was to develop a method which could be applied to most if not all transradial levels, allow the prosthesis to be worn as long as necessary from day 1 and maximise residual forearm flexion. The SSOS utilises the area above the olecranon on the triceps tendon as the main suspension area. Parallel medial and lateral 'wings' extend over the epicondyles. The primary purpose of these extensions is to keep the posterior

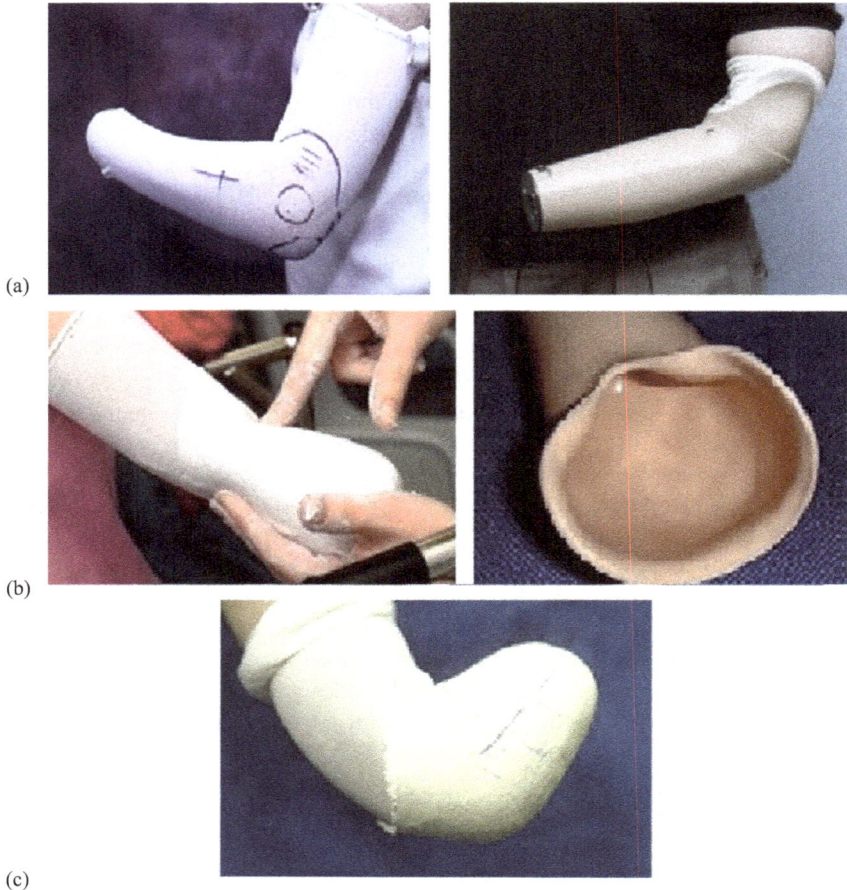

Figure 2.5   Examples of SSOS (a), Muenster socket (b), Brim socket plaster cast (c)

section of the socket in place rather than to provide suspension, as the area above the epicondyles does not have a good tolerance to pressure. The anterior of the socket is the only trimline that varies depending on stump length.

The Otto Bock socket is a tight-fitting socket that cups the olecranon and epicondyles using a combination of indirect skeletal suspension and tissue restriction to provide suspension. Due to its intimate fit, a distal pull-in tube is usually required for donning.

The three-fourths of the socket was developed in response to feedback from patients that their arms got too hot in the tight-fitting sockets required for myoelectric control. Through an analysis of the below-elbow socket, Sauter *et al.* determined that the proximal posterior quadrant which covers the elbow had no functional purpose, and so a socket design evolved with this area cut-away. Reported benefits

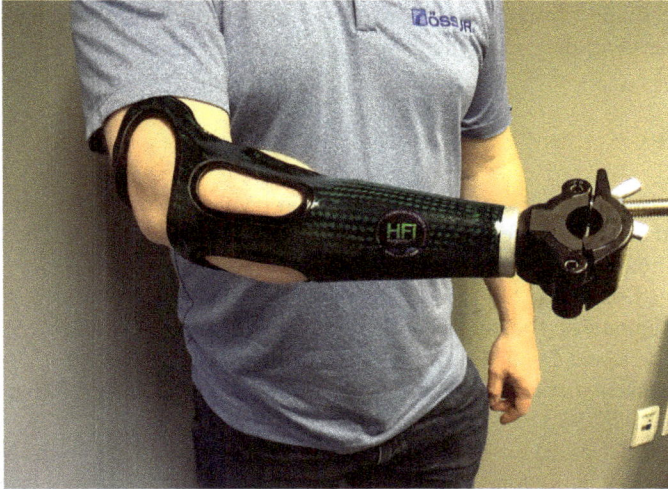

Figure 2.6   TR prosthesis with Hi-Fi socket

include increased ventilation and improved suspension secondary to decreased perspiration.

The WILMER is an open socket design by Dick Plettenburg from Delft University. Unlike traditional total contact designs, the WILMER is constructed using stainless steel tubing which is covered with a cushioned fabric. Advantages of this system are increased ventilation for the residual limb and skin contact with the external environment. Tissues, however, are not stabilised and stump socket forces may be higher due to the non-total-contact design.

The Hi-Fi interface (Hi-Fi socket) designed by Randall Alley is a patented design based on the compression-release stabilisation theory. This socket design differs from previous sockets as its primary goal is that of skeletal control rather than limb accommodation and containment. An alternating array of longitudinally shaped compression areas in distinct locations, as shown in Figure 2.6, coupled with release zones form a denser matrix of soft tissue around the bone, restricting its motion, creating improved stability, and a reported better linkage between the wearer and prosthesis. Patients provide feedback on compression levels during casting/scanning and throughout the process to ensure desired function and comfort.

2.6   Conclusion

The importance of the socket is often overlooked when considering advances in prosthetic technology. If the prosthesis is to become truly integrated into the wearer's life then the design of the socket, including how it has been fabricated, must be customised to their individual needs. There may come a time soon when we are able to automate parts of the shape capture, modification and fabrication processes, but ultimately socket success will determine the comfort and function of the device.

References

[1]   Davidson J. A survey of the satisfaction of upper limb amputees with their prostheses, their lifestyles, and their abilities. Journal of Hand Therapy. 2002; 15(1):62–70.

[2]   Kejlaa GH. Consumer concerns and the functional value of prostheses to upper limb amputees. Prosthetics and Orthotics International. 1993;17(3):157–163.

[3]   Biddiss E and Chau T. Upper-limb prosthetics: critical factors in device abandonment. American Journal of Physical Medicine and Rehabilitation. 2007; 86(12):977–987.

[4]   Kyberd PJ and Hill W. Survey of upper limb prosthesis users in Sweden, the United Kingdom and Canada. Prosthetics and Orthotics International. 2011;35(2):234–241.

[5]   Millstein SG, Heger H, and Hunter GA. Prosthetic use in adult upper limb amputees: a comparison of the body powered and electrically powered prostheses. Prosthetics and Orthotics International. 1986;10(1):27–34.

[6]   Mak AF, Zhang M, and Boone DA. State-of-the-art research in lower-limb prosthetic biomechanics-socket interface: a review. Journal of Rehabilitation Research and Development. 2001;38(2):161–174.

[7]   Bader DL and Worsley PR. Technologies to monitor the health of loaded skin tissues. Biomedical Engineering Online. 2018;17(1):40.

[8]   Dumbleton T, Buis AWP, McFadyen A, *et al.* Dynamic interface pressure distributions of two transtibial prosthetic socket concepts. Journal of Rehabilitation Research and Development. 2009;46(3):405–415.

[9]   Gefen A, Farid KJ, and Shaywitz I. A review of deep tissue injury development, detection, and prevention: shear savvy. Ostomy Wound Management. 2013;59(2):26–35.

[10]   Graser M, Day S, and Buis AWP. Exploring the role of transtibial prosthetic use in deep tissue injury development: a scoping review. BMC Biomedical Engineering. 2020;2:2.

[11]   Day S and Wands-Silva K. Opinions of paediatric upper limb amputees. In: Myoelectric Control Symposium (MEC'14); 2014. p. 1.

[12]   Twiste M. Limbless statistics: a repository for quantitative information on the UK limbless population REFERRED for prosthetics treatment: annual report 2010–2011. University of Salford; 2013. Available from: http://www.limbless-statistics.org/.

Chapter 3

Methods for clinical evaluation

*Laurence Kenney[1], Peter Kyberd[2], Adam Galpin[1],
Alix Chadwell[1], Malcolm Granat[1], Sibylle Thies[1]
and John Head[1]*

Techniques for the evaluation of upper limb prostheses have developed over many decades, driven by advances in prosthetic technology and technologies for their assessment, as well as our understanding of human motor control, psychology and, most recently, real-world behaviours. The upper limb is not just a functional tool; it is used to communicate, is used to show emotion and indeed plays a key role in our sense of who we are. Therefore, replacement of part, or all, of an upper limb by an artificial device, no matter how sophisticated, leads to not only changes in our abilities to pick up and manipulate objects, but also how we interact with the world in other ways. This chapter provides the reader with an overview of the methods and tools available to characterise these behaviours, both with a view to evaluating the prostheses themselves and the effectiveness of the methods used to train users.

It is worth considering from the outset the kind of information that different groups might want from an evaluation. Clinicians sometimes frame their evaluations in the World Health Organisation (WHO) International Classification of Functioning, Disability and Health (ICF) [1]. The ICF considers human functioning to sit in four areas: 'body functions and structures', 'activities and participation', 'environmental factors' and 'personal factors'. This structure is designed to be applicable across different health domains and is very clearly focused on the experience of users themselves, aimed at clinicians who want to understand how to make a patient's life better. Many of the traditional outcome measures fit neatly into this structure [2]. Design engineers may take a different perspective on the evaluation, favouring measures which provide objective information which is of value to their goal of producing better prostheses. Although outcome measures used in this context may also fit within the ICF, the engineers may also want additional (device-specific) information to help interpret the observations of the participant's behaviours. Finally, motor control scientists may be interested in how a user's interaction with an artificial limb can help unpick underlying motor and psychological processes and hence inform training regimes. The process of selecting an appropriate set of outcome measures is therefore likely to be influenced

[1]Centre for Health Sciences Research, University of Salford, Salford, UK
[2]School of Energy and Electronic Engineering, University of Portsmouth, Portsmouth, UK

by the domain within which the design engineer, researcher or clinician is working, and this aspect is discussed in more detail later in this chapter. This chapter does not aim to comprehensively review all the available tools, rather it focuses on a broad introduction to the different approaches to evaluation. The reader is directed to other texts at relevant parts of this chapter for more information.

This chapter begins with an introduction to the challenges of measurement in upper limb prosthetics. This is followed by an overview of the traditional approaches to evaluation and their strengths and weaknesses. By traditional approaches, we mean tests involving observation of a participant performing a structured activity or reporting on their everyday experiences and behaviours through questionnaires. These approaches generally involve little, if any, instrumentation and are still widely used. In the next section, we report on the evaluation tools which have emerged from studies of human motor control; these include observation of the kinematics during the performance of tasks and measures which may reflect attentional demands, such as gaze behaviours and brain activity. As the so-called conventional methods and the human-motor-control-based methods either observe behaviours over a short period of time or ask people to accurately recall and report on their behaviours, both have inherent limitations. Finally, we report on methods which can be used to capture, in detail, the everyday upper limb behaviours of people in the real world and discuss the opportunities such real-world approaches open up around data analysis at scale.

3.1   Measurement issues in upper limb prosthetics

Before going on to discuss the various approaches to the evaluation of upper limb prostheses, it is worth considering a few key issues. First, a good outcome test can be used by different persons on different days and in different places, on the same subject, and the results should be comparable. If the measurement changes, then change recorded should be meaningful. This presents a challenge in the creation of a test, which is at the same time meaningful and comparable. Fundamental to the problem of evaluation of upper limb prostheses is the characteristic that hands and arms are capable of a very wide range of operations, for a wide range of purposes. Even with a prosthetic limb with fewer motions and a more limited control format, the operators can be very imaginative in finding effective solutions to problems so that it is difficult to create a single test that easily captures the full value of a prosthesis to the individual. Moreover, comparing one imaginative solution to another is hard. Conversely, if a test involves observing a subject carrying out a single simple operation (such as timing someone to pick up an object), it is easy to make a comparison between performances. The test can produce simple unambiguous numbers (e.g. range of motion, time to complete, force imparted), which can be easily understood. However, the results of such tests may be of very limited value to the clinician, the engineer or the motor-control expert; for example, how does the speed with which someone can pick up an object from a horizontal surface relate to how well they can use their device in their daily life?

If, instead, the test involves some complex actions that more reflect user experience, then there may be as many solutions to the test as subjects taking it and so comparisons would have to be vague and descriptive. Thus, the design of a useful test is a compromise between ease of interpretation and depth of information about the capabilities of the user. The traditional outcome measures have generally sat somewhere on the spectrum from simple but limited in range to complex but hard to interpret. The examples of methods in the rest of this chapter show different solutions to this problem and towards the end, discuss the potential for recently introduced real-world evaluation to deliver on both fronts.

3.2 Traditional methods

The ICF was developed by the WHO [3,4] and was released in 2001. Its aims were to create a language for all of the health professions to be able to unambiguously describe the health status of any person. Its emphasis was on the individual. This meant that it looked at the person's ability to function and not on their disability. It aimed to create a parity between impairments. So instead of talking about impairments, activity limitations or handicaps, it divided the world into three domains: Body Structures and Functions, Activity and Participation. Once classified simply, it would then be easier to identify ways to assist or overcome the limitations that society's structures imposed on the individual.

A group of professionals in upper limb prosthetics (Upper Limb Prosthetics Outcome Measures Group) adopted this model to describe the different needs for assessment [5,6]. Just as it is impossible to measure the speed or acceleration of a car and the enjoyment that driving the car gives the owner, with the same single question. It is not possible to measure the performance, the functional capabilities of a device and how a person actually uses it. So, the domains were taken as the driver for each of the categories of assessment:

Function. Simple measures of performance of the prosthesis mechanism, such as the speed of opening or the grip strength. These are things that can be measured with simple devices (stopwatch, strain gauge, etc.).

Activity. What the person can do with the prosthesis. Usually measured using standardised activities in the lab and observing or timing their performance.

Participation. What the person actually does with the device. This was previously measured using surveys or questionnaires. These methods are limited and have numerous flaws. Any respondent is unlikely to be objective or have a good memory for details. This is true for all surveys, in any circumstance, not just prosthesis users. Asking someone how much alcohol they drink in an average week rarely nets an accurate measure. What is recorded may be larger or smaller depending on who is asking the questions. Newer and potentially more accurate measures have been developed and are described next.

3.2.1 Questionnaires – participation domain

Until very recently questionnaires were the only way to assess the users' perspective of a device. More modern direct observation techniques, such as head-mounted cameras and activity monitors, are now possible as an adjunct to a survey (see later).

It can be difficult to ensure that a survey or questionnaire is useful. It is important to make sure that the wording is carefully designed to be unambiguous, easily understood, and so as not to lead a respondent to answer in a particular direction, biasing the result.

The first aspect a questionnaire must address is to make it understandable by the intended audience. If there is a language or education bias, using words or phrases that the audience cannot understand or will misinterpret, then only some of the population will respond meaningfully, or at all. Short and quick surveys are more easily answered. Longer words with subtle meaning that take time to interpret can easily put off respondents and such a bias will mean any conclusion drawn from the results is based on only parts of the population (people who have a lot of time or are persistent) and so not generally applicable.

The next concern is that the questions are culturally appropriate. Activities with one hand (left or right) are distinctly different, depending on the practices of a user's culture. It is not simply a matter of dominant and non-dominant but also depends upon acceptable activities within a culture or group. For example, which hand do you use to attend to your toilet? Questions of utility such as this can have entirely different answers depending on custom and practice. Similarly, what is the language used? If the questionnaire was written in one language, then the translation of a questionnaire into a different language is not trivial. It cannot be performed by one person who has a good grasp on the local dialect. The proper understanding of the subtleties of use is paramount. Therefore, the only way to check the correct translation is to get one person to translate into the language and an entirely independent person to transform it back to the original language. If what comes back is not precisely what the question setter meant, then there is something wrong with the translation. It is too easy to miss intent with a language, to mean something subtle and different to what a non-native might mean. This was why when the Americans and the Soviets first worked together in space in a joint mission in 1976, the Americans spoke in Russian and the Russians spoke in American. Space is a dangerous environment and misunderstandings can be fatal. Only then could they be sure that the meaning was 'by the book'.

A final consideration is the length of the questionnaire. If it is long and daunting, then subjects may not start or complete it. Modern life is full of attempts to measure the quality of service. Most of them based around consumer concerns are biased towards the product. The vendor can entice the subject towards completion through inducements (e.g. prize draws, credits on the next purchase). A properly constructed and unbiased survey may not be as engaging and may be less likely to be completed if it does not quickly get to the point. When the author PJK designed a questionnaire for people who attended the Oxford Limb centre, the original aim was a single side of paper. In the end, it expanded to four pages but enjoyed a response rate of nearly 70%.

3.2.2   Observational measures – activity domain

The ability of an experienced observer to be able to detect subtleties in movement may be as yet unsurpassed. In prosthetic use therapists are able to see the smallest changes to movement to accommodate limitations in the prosthesis. The drawback is the need to have considerable experience before reliable and precise measures are possible. Generally, such tests must be conducted by an experienced observer, trained to observe the prosthesis user in a particular way. To achieve this, the design must also be carefully made.

3.2.2.1 Assessment of Capacity of Myoelectric Control

The Assessment of Capacity of Myoelectric Control (ACMC) [7,8] is a tool designed by Liselotte Hermansson from the Orebro clinic in Sweden. Its name is very precise and reflects its careful design.

The ACMC attempts to get around the one of the major flaws in the design of many tests. The ideal test results in a wide spread of scores from low to high. Most tests are either too hard so that most will get a very low mark (a floor) or so easy that too many of the subjects will end up with full marks (a ceiling). In both the instances, little can be said about those subjects. With a limit, they may all be as good, but more likely there is a range and the measurement has failed to detect it. A more carefully designed tool would get around this. The ACMC was based on a career of experience of guiding users to improve their function. Other tests could separate the weak from the strong but could not incorporate the most talented. An example is one of Hermansson's colleagues, who could tie a bow behind her back using one standard myo hand (no additional feedback) and one natural hand. She would be up against the ceiling in any other test.

A second flaw in most tests is that everyone designs their life around how they solve certain routine problems, for example, always approaching an object and problem from one angle. For the fully able this is almost invisible, but anyone who does the same task often will tend to perform it the same way, even if there are different ways to achieve the same goal. When reduction in performance happens, people have to ensure that they find effective ways to solve routine problems. This is true for impairments of motor or sensory control (motor neurone disease or Parkinson's) or a reduction in the number of working joints, such as amputation. In each case, the individuals will find a way to solve that particular problem, and may become proficient at their own, sometimes unique approach, over time.

Activity domain tests consist of activities or simulated activities that are observed, recorded or timed. If those activities are routine, the person will not need to learn the task and will simply perform it to the best of their ability. If the task is new, what the test does is examine the person's ability to adapt to a new circumstance, a worthy topic of study. But it is not the same as determining the ability of the subject. So, a test that has one subject used to a task (and so is proficient) and one who is learning as they do it does not create an accurate comparison between them.

The ACMC is designed differently. It asks a subject to perform a task they are familiar with and then observes how they solve it. So, if the user opted to make a cake, they would have to go into a kitchen, search for the correct tools (spoons, bowls, ingredients), bring them together and prepare the cake. The observer would then see how they went about the task. For example, when they searched for the bowl, they would need to open cupboards. Do they open them only with the sound hand (if they have one)? Or do they open two together with both hands? When they pick up an object, if it is on the prosthetic side, do they use the prosthesis? Or do they reach across their body with their sound hand and pick it up? Then do they pick it up with the sound hand, do they carry it in that hand or press it into the prosthesis to carry? All of these actions are scored together and combined to give the subject a score. During the design of the tool, Hermansson compared results using Rasch analysis to weight the scores of different activities to ensure no floors or ceilings in the range.

Thus, the ACMC was designed and tests showed that the most reproducible results came from therapists of long experience. However, it is worth noting that the point about the test is to allow the assessor to see more precisely how a device is used. Therefore, a prosthetist or design engineer may benefit from learning to administer the test which, in turn, may help them to see the world a little more like a highly skilled OT.

ACMC was launched in 2008 and has been used in many centres. It is currently NOT appropriate to use it to assess the function of a person with a body-powered device, although undoubtedly it would give the observer significant insight if they observed activities in this manner. At the time of writing, there are moves in Orebro to produce a body-powered variant. We await it with interest.

3.2.3   Time-based outcome measures – activity domain

One of the simplest measures of performance is the time taken. One can argue that the faster a person performs a task the more control they have in its execution. It is common to question this as a metric for prosthetic function. This is to misunderstand the reasoning behind its use. As stated before, the measurement of some aspect of performance can be a surrogate for that performance. So, speed of operation does not just measure how fast a person can perform a task, it also measures how good their control of a prosthesis is, and how able the prosthesis is at performing the task. It provides a repeatable measure that is easy to record, although as discussed earlier, it does not capture many other elements of prosthesis control.

3.2.3.1   The Southampton Hand Assessment Procedure

The Southampton Hand Assessment Procedure (SHAP) was designed by Light and Chappell in the response to the fact that there were no simple unambiguous tools to measure prosthetic function [9,10]. Southampton University was pioneer in the computer control of prosthetic hands, including creating the first microprocessor-controlled field used prosthetic limb. The team needed to demonstrate that combining a more sophisticated control format and a multi-axis hand could change the functional capabilities of the user. So Light created a tool in the activity domain that measured how a hand was used by performing a range of simulated activities of daily living (ADLs). A study as part of the design phase showed that busy clinics would not use all of any of the existing tests (such as the Jebsen–Taylor test [11]), because it took too long to complete. Some clinics took a shortcut and would use only part of the Jebsen–Taylor test, rendering the results without merit outside that individual's experience. The therapist could use her/his experience and employ it as an observational tool, but without validation the results were meaningless to outsiders. In response to this, SHAP was designed to be simple and quick to administer so that it could be used in a clinic, and its results were shared and understood more widely.

SHAP consists of a form board, a timer and a series of activities which simulate ADLs (Figure 3.1). As there are many ways to perform a task, the role of the SHAP kit constrains the task to one that can be performed repeatedly and in a reasonable time in a busy clinic.

The form board constrains the activity to a limited envelope and solutions to the problem so that it is easy to compare two persons performing the activity. The timer is started and stopped by the subject. This removes the uncertainty that an external timer would introduce; when has the person started? The ADLs were chosen from the literature and were seen to be those that were most consistent when used to measure human performance and reflected a range of tasks that would be representative of the sorts of actions a person might wish to undertake with the hand.

The choices were made to make the test as repeatable as possible. The tasks were divided into two groups: abstract objects. Twelve objects (two sets of six, light and heavy) were designed to be manipulated by six canonical grasps (Tips, Extension, Lateral, Tripod, Spherical and Cylindrical). These objects were picked up from one defined position on the form board and placed on another; simulated ADLs. Fourteen tasks designed to need to be performed by the full range of grasps. Start and stop positions are defined by marks on the form board.

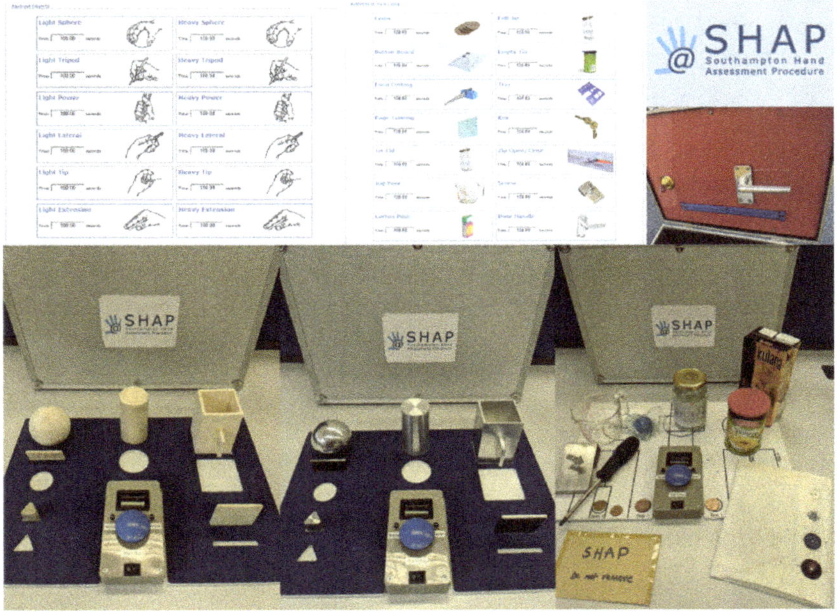

Figure 3.1   Southampton Hand Assessment Procedure

The test runs through all tasks using the hand under test (the prosthesis) as the dominant hand. Scoring is based on the difference between the time recorded by the subject and that of a nominal group of standard subjects. The final value is not a simple mean but is weighted by the (assumed real world) frequency of use of the grasp employed. So an uncommonly used grasp pattern will have less impact on the score than a common one. The philosophy is to explore the practical functionality of the hand, so a task that requires a Lateral grip, but can be performed by a different grasp still counts, but will still be scored as if it was a Lateral grip and still will have less an impact on the overall assessment.

The SHAP aims to measure the functional performance of the hand under test, not the person themselves. For this reason, the same person with a different prosthesis would get a different score. SHAP was also aimed at being used in a wider range of impairments than simply upper limb prosthetics. For example, it could be used to assess natural hand functionality before and after injury and during rehabilitation.

The SHAP has been validated not only by the originating team but by others in the field (hence an additional air of objectivity) [12]. It has been used by many different research groups as one of a suite of assessments when measuring new prosthesis designs. This is very much the correct use of the tool, as part of a range of tests to get the full picture. In summary, SHAP establishes a simple framework that can be used as the basis of other protocols. It removes the need for a team to devise and validate a new test, simply to integrate the supplementary protocol.

However, it is not uncommon for some researchers to criticise SHAP for what it cannot do, or how it determines a functionality score. One concern is that time is used as a metric and some commenters are concerned that this is not how users generally employ their devices. This is true, but as this is a test the users will tend to try and complete the task as fast as they can without undue strain. Additionally, the speed of operation reflects the ease of control and the functionality of the design. Simply put, if it is easier to use then it will be used more quickly. This is supported by independent assessment of SHAP which showed that the functional performance was closely associated with time to completion [13].

A second concern is that most persons with a single side loss will not habitually use their devices in this way. Both of these concerns fundamentally misinterpret the aim of the design of the tool. This is a tool aimed at activity domain. It looks at the way a hand could be used, not how it is used. By controlling the measurements, comparisons are possible. If someone wishes to know more about how a hand is used, the clinician needs to employ a measure of the participation domain. It is wrong to expect SHAP to measure user satisfaction or daily use as it is designed specifically to measure activity. Finally, some researchers have raised the issue of a learning effect over multiple repeats, and the opaque scoring system, proposing an alternative [14,15].

3.2.4   Clinic-based activities

There are a few tests that have emerged from the clinic, adapted from training tools that have been liked by the occupational therapists, and their use has been standardised to give a recognised tool. A couple of examples of these are discussed next.

3.2.4.1 Box and blocks

This is a standard manipulation tool that involves subjects picking up one block from many in a tray, moving it over a barrier to a second tray (both lids of the carrying box) and dropping it in the other side [16]. This is a simple activity that requires the user to be able to grasp a single block of a random orientation in a precision grip and then raise it more than 10 cm and laterally more than this, before releasing it. The task therefore involves a number of coordinated moves that a prosthesis user should be able to do. The blocks are all in front of the subject and only around the mid line. If the subject has less range of motion and has to move her/his body left and right rather than use humeral deviation to move from one attempt to the other, this becomes clear to the observer, making it a useful evaluation tool.

As a training exercise, the limitations of range and space are not particularly important, nor is the fact that if all the blocks supplied are placed in the box, they will be packed so tightly in the base that extracting them becomes difficult for the fully able. Similarly, the orientation and position of the blocks mean that the time to pick up a block varies greatly, making the time poorly controlled.

Numerous variations of the B&B have therefore been proposed:

- Limiting the number of blocks while having them randomly resting in the box.
- Placing a few blocks in a defined grid pattern with a set order means that it can be used with motion tracking technology and the different actions directly compared.

An additional variation is to use fragile object rather than wooden blocks so that 'egg and box' tests have been used to compare manipulative performance with touch feedback [17].

3.2.4.2 Clothespin Relocation Task

A second training tool that has been adopted into clinical measurement is the Clothespin Relocation Task [18–20]. This consists of a simple apparatus with a vertical and a horizontal rod and a series of spring clothes pegs, with different spring rates. The task is to move pegs from the horizontal to the vertical rod and back. It requires the user to perform precision grips in positions from the middle of the body, rotate the peg and be able to release the peg when it is high up and the arm is at full stretch. This wide range of motion may mean that a voluntary opening, body-powered terminal device (TD) may not release at full stretch (or the peg may fall from the grasp in a voluntary closing TD). Conversely, a transradial myoelectric socket may not allow the elbow to fully extend, as limits on elbow flexion due to the socket are common in self-suspending sockets. The higher reach needed when interacting with pegs on the vertical rod may also put the socket in a position where the user cannot generate a clear signal to open the hand to grasp or release the peg.

One really useful aspect of the test is that the TD must be rotated from horizontal to vertical orientation to complete the task. If the operator employs corrective motions at the shoulder to achieve this, rather than to operate the prosthetic wrist to pro/supinate the hand, this is clearly evident to both subject and assessor, without the need for motion capture equipment. Thus, it is a useful test for prostheses which offer more than one degree of freedom, and it was originally made into an assessment tool by

Kathy Stubblefield of the RIC team in Chicago as they investigated the impact of targeted muscle reinnervation as a procedure [19].

The limitations in the use of the standard device include the fact that the basic equipment is not symmetrical (the rod is only on one side of the base) meaning that results differ between left-side and right-side operation. Additionally, the position of the pegs at the start or at the end was not standardised, meaning that the order could potentially change the timing of the total activity.

Hussaini has worked on a standardised protocol with a modification to the equipment to make it symmetrical and an order of the pegs. Initial work involved using motion capture techniques to quantify body movement corrections. This level of equipment and testing time is inappropriate in the clinic so he abstracted the work into a purely time and observational tool that would allow a person to be assessed in a matter of minutes and give usable results [18,20,21].

3.2.4.3 Activities measure for upper limb amputees

Historically, tests were devised by individuals in local centres and there was little or no attempt to validate the tools or measure the psychometric properties of a tool. From 2000 onwards, this began to change with attempts to take a more structured approach to outcome measure design. One of the results of this approach is the Activities Measure for Upper Limb Amputees (AM-ULA), developed by Linda Resnik as part of the US DARPA prosthetic arm program [22]. The aim of the program was to produce a prosthetic system with a greater number of degrees of freedom than is routinely used. The resulting hand raised some of the same concerns about evaluation that Light *et al.* had encountered in Southampton decades earlier [10], i.e. a need for a tool that tests the device's capabilities sufficiently.

The designers of AM-ULA sought to create a valid tool with good psychometric properties, in the activity domain. It is based around a series of simulated ADLs and is scored by a trained observer and activity timing. The test is scored between 0 and 40 (the higher value relates to higher performance) and is based on the following elements: the extent of completion of subtasks, the speed of completion, movement quality, skill of prosthetic use and independence. The test is based on 18 tasks chosen for the test based on those which showed inter-rater validity (test-rest ICC > 0.5). Its validity was demonstrated by comparing with other existing tests, establishing convergent validity. The test proved to be too long for all circumstances, so more recently the team has worked to make it quicker to deliver (while retaining its psychometric properties), the Brief AM-ULA [23].

3.3 Laboratory-based techniques

This section introduces evaluation tools which have emerged from studies of human motor control carried out under controlled conditions (hence the term 'laboratory-based techniques'). They are grounded in an understanding of what constitutes normal patterns of upper limb motor control and the characteristic deviations from this which appear when studying people using prosthetic limbs. Some of the approaches described here may not be sufficiently mature/developed to use as evaluation tools but do point to future potential ways of extending our understanding of how to evaluate prostheses. The section begins with an overview of gaze behaviours, followed by a section on kinematics, and finally a section on the emerging area of brain activity behaviours during prosthesis use.

As discussed by Bongers *et al.* [24], there are several fundamental ways in which upper limb motor control using a prosthesis is more challenging than motor control for anatomically intact people. The main issues can be summarised as follows:

1. **Control**. In all cases, prostheses are controlled in a way which differs significantly from the equivalent in anatomically intact people. In the case of body-powered prostheses, control of hand opening/closing comes from movement of the contralateral shoulder and is further complicated by mechanical coupling of hand activation to the configurations of the distal joints (Chadwell – in preparation). There are also a small number of semi-passive devices, which may be opened or closed using the contralateral limb, or by pressing against objects in the environment; clearly neither example is close to replicating normal prehension. In the case of myoelectric prostheses, the mapping from the measured EMG signal to the dynamics of the hand is inevitably constrained by the amount of information that can be extracted from sites, the signal processing approaches taken and the number of motors and their dynamics. Further, most clinical devices use socket-located electrodes, and therefore small shifts in the socket introduce uncertainty into the controller in the form of motion artefacts, and/or loss of contact between the electrode and skin. Such issues can lead to unwanted activations, or frustration with the prosthesis not responding to the user's commands [25,26].

2. **Sensory feedback**. Although there are some impressive advances in the field [27,28], the vast majority of myoelectric prostheses offer no feedback to the user. A degree of feedback on force and aperture is available to users of body-powered devices via tension in the control cable and postural configuration; however, this may not be intuitive to interpret.

3. **Mechanical degrees of freedom**. All current body-powered devices and, until around 2010, the commercially available myoelectric prostheses, offer(ed) only a single degree of freedom prehensor. Although multi-articulated hands have, as the name implies, many mechanical joints, the number of controllable, independent degrees of freedom is small. This inevitably leads to constraints on how objects are approached, acquired and manipulated. Such constraints are often accommodated by adjustments to more proximal joint trajectories.

Given these challenges, it is unsurprising that patterns of motor control exhibited by users of upper limb prostheses differ from the norm. Measurements of speed and accuracy alone do not provide detailed information about online aspects of performance such as kinematics or the ongoing allocation of visual attention. Self-report on task performance must necessarily be done retrospectively because asking users to simultaneously report on behaviour impacts on their cognitive resources and affects ongoing performance.

Therefore, in this section we will review laboratory-based techniques which afford analysis of aspects of prosthesis control which are not amenable to self-report or simple performance measures. For instance, eye-tracking techniques allow fine-grained insight into visuomotor control strategies employed during task completion. Kinematic measurement affords analysis of motor performance variables, including limb segment trajectories, joint angles and grip force. Measures of neural activity provide indices of mental effort. Importantly, these techniques produce temporally rich, objective, data that can be used to compare performance between users (individuals or groups), as well as across time. Such data offers insight into the trajectory of motor learning and the characteristics of prosthesis expertise, in addition to the aspects of task performance which present the greatest challenges for prosthesis users. Finally, techniques such as this offer valuable information for designers, providing insight into underlying mechanisms by which a given hand may or may not be supporting a user's performance.

3.3.1   Gaze behaviour

Detailed visual information is limited to the central (foveal) 2 degrees of the human visual field. Consequently, we need to move our eyes, head or trunk in order to extract rich visual information from the environment. Researchers can therefore obtain insight into what area of the visual world an observer is currently processing by measuring where their eyes are oriented. Eye-tracking is a technique that calibrates the direction of gaze with locations in the visual world. The earliest eye-tracking technology required fitting a device directly to an observer's eyeball, but modern techniques are far less invasive. Video-based eye-tracking shines a safe infrared light into the eyes and detects the reflection of this light on the cornea, in addition to identifying the pupil. The relative position of the pupil and corneal reflection changes as the eye rotates in the socket allowing detection of where the eyes are pointing. Gaze recording usually begins with a calibration process which requires the participant to systematically fixate different points across the area of the visual field of interest in the research. Once completed, this allows an eye-tracking system to map the rotation of the eyeball to different points in space and infer the focus of gaze.

Advances in this technology now mean that the necessary hardware can be contained on a lightweight head-mounted device (see [29], for a recent review of head-mounted eye-tracker technology). These devices often resemble a pair of glasses which contain a scene camera for filming what is in front of an observer and one or two eye cameras which record the eyes. Employing this technology allows an observer to move around their environment and complete tasks in three-dimensional space. At the same time, a data file is collected which overlays an eye fixation point over a video of the observer's visual world. Most head-mounted systems have dedicated calibration procedures built into their software, consisting of one or more points which are presented to the researcher on the scene view and then aligned to a detail in the real world which the participant must then fixate. When designing activities, it should be considered that eye-tracking is most accurate for objects in the same depth plane as the calibration points, although most systems are able to compensate for some of this 'parallax error' [29].

Data analysis of the video output depends on the requirement of the particular study, but typical analyses will often consider when, how long and how often certain areas of interest (AoIs) are fixated. For instance, as described next, relevant AoIs for reaching and grasping studies include the hand, the target of the reach and any additional objects relevant to future phases of the action. Computing gaze parameters for AoIs is straightforward when eye-tracking two-dimensional static images and involves simply providing coordinates for the boundaries of the AoI. Dedicated analysis software can then provide data on eye behaviour for each AoI. However, processing eye data from real-world activities is considerably more challenging because the output is a video and the position of an AoI within the scene is dynamic due to participant head movements. Coordinates cannot be used for such data, and therefore, a common (and time-consuming) approach is to code the fixation location frame-by-frame. Efforts to automatically code objects within videos have been made, but these are less reliable than manual coding because automatic systems are unable to make sensible decisions in instances when fixation location is ambiguous. One such instance could be when one AoI passes in front of another, or when fixation is on a boundary between two AoIs. Therefore, researchers are often required to develop complex 'coding schemes' incorporating multiple AoIs, rules for resolving ambiguities and use of two or more coders to test inter-rate reliability [30]. Figure 3.2 shows an example of data collected with an eye tracker and the resultant coded data.

One last consideration for designing studies employing head-mounted eye-trackers involves where the activities take place relative to the body. When people manipulate objects very close to their trunk (such as using a mobile phone), their eyes are directed downwards and the eye-lids obscure most of the eye from the eye cameras. This problem is more severe when the cameras are fixed within the frames of eye-tracking glasses but is still a problem even with those eye-trackers where the eye cameras are adjustable. It is therefore sensible to arrange task-relevant objects on

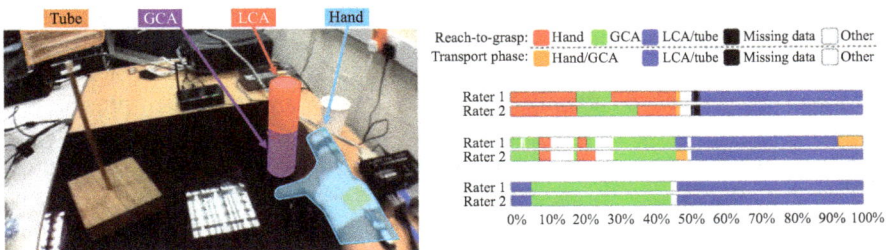

Figure 3.2   *Example screenshot of video data from a scene camera in an eye-tracker (left), together with an example of coded gaze behaviour. Here the scene is divided into a set of AoIs, in this case tube, grasp critical area (GCA), location critical area (LCA) and other (left). For each video frame, the location of the gaze with respect to the set of AoIs is coded, allowing for graphical representation of the gaze over time (right)*

a table top that is quite high relative to the participant's trunk and at such a distance that their eyes are directed forwards and not down. Combined with the recommendation to keep the whole activity within the same depth plane, this means that there is unavoidable artificiality in many of the tasks designed for head-mounted eye-trackers.

Researchers in other fields have measured how observers allocate their visual attention across a range of activities, including familiar everyday tasks such as making a cup of tea [31] or hand washing [32]. Studies have also compared performance of experts versus novices in highly skilled tasks such as performing laparoscopic surgery [33]. Several key findings from this literature are relevant to understanding eye-tracking studies of visuomotor control in prosthesis use. First, eye fixations during familiar tasks are focused overwhelmingly on objects or areas of space relevant for task completion ('top-down' factors) and are rarely driven by the visual salience of objects ('bottom-up' factors). Second, eye fixation locations during reaching and grasping follow a stereotyped pattern whereby gaze anchors the reach target (e.g. a bottle) and then moves to subsequent objects (e.g. a wine glass) as the hand makes contact, or shortly before [34]. Third, gaze becomes increasingly predictive (i.e. looking ahead to the end point of an action) as a novel task becomes familiar [35]. Fourth, during very familiar tasks, gaze may 'look ahead' to objects relevant to future components of a task [32]. Fifth, during tool use, gaze switches between the target and the tool in novices but is fixated on the target in experts [33]. Such a body of literature lays the foundations for the predictions that have driven the eye-tracking studies in prosthesis users. In such studies, an expert pattern of gaze has been assumed to involve an anchoring of gaze to the target of an action and not directed to the prosthesis itself. Novice use is assumed to involve increased visual monitoring of the prosthetic hand, which may also involve frequent switches between the hand and target objects. Very skilled users may require less mental effort for ongoing actions and can therefore afford to 'look ahead' to future task components.

Laboratory studies on eye-tracking and prosthesis use have attempted to understand the pattern of gaze in both prosthesis users [13,36–38] and anatomically intact participants fitted with a prosthesis simulator over their anatomical arm and hand [36,39,40]. The advantage of using the simulator is that it allows skill acquisition to be analysed in a controlled setting and can increase access to research participants. However, assessing real prosthesis users offers insight into the visuomotor strategies that have been developed naturally to maximise performance with their prosthesis.

In the first eye-tracking study of prosthesis users, Bouwsema *et al.* [13] analysed gaze performance in 5 (relatively experienced) prosthesis users who were required to pick up a non-familiar compressible object over 40 trials. The findings indicated variable gaze behaviour whereby some users mostly fixated the object, while some switched frequently between fixating the object and the hand. The authors noted that use of the 'switching' pattern corresponded with those who reported less use of the prosthesis in the real world. However, it did not correspond well with functional skill level. Importantly, neither relationship was investigated statistically. Sobuh *et al.* [36] studied four prosthesis uses and seven anatomically intact users who were learning to control a prosthesis simulator during a pouring task (lifting a carton and pouring into a glass). The focus of this study was on gaze behaviour across the learning trajectory, and therefore, the simulator users were analysed over three training sessions. The study also included a baseline task, whereby the simulator users first completed the task with their intact limb. While the baseline task showed the expected fixation bias towards the target objects, gaze behaviour with the use of the simulator showed frequent switches between the hand and the object and a reliance on fixating the hand. An example of the gaze data from Sobuh's study is given in Figure 3.3.

Training had no statistical effect on this pattern. One interpretation is that three training sessions were not enough for users to develop the expected pattern of gaze. However, the four experienced prosthesis users, who had chance to develop the expected gaze behaviour through extensive practice, showed strikingly similar results to those using the prosthesis simulator. The reliance on fixation on the prosthetic hand compared to a healthy hand was also found by Parr *et al.* [39] with a larger sample of 21 users of a prosthesis simulator. Participants were required to drag coins across a table before picking them up and placing them in a container (derived from SHAP). In the largest study of gaze behaviour in prosthesis users to date ($n = 20$), Chadwell

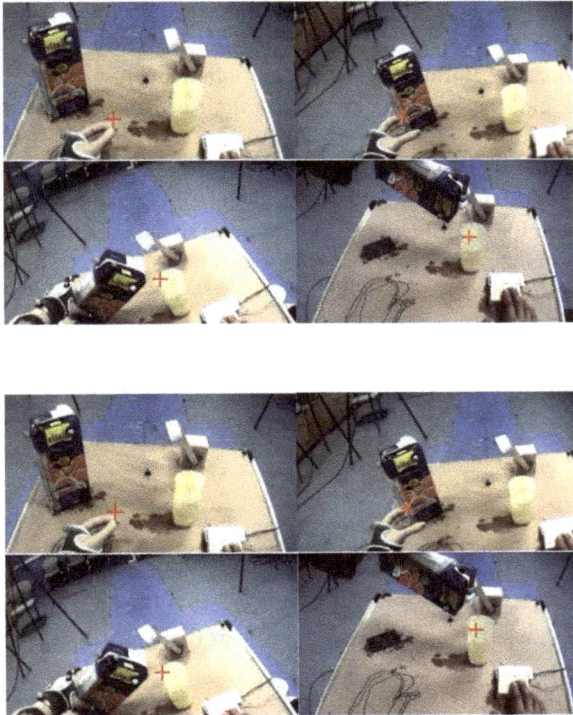

Figure 3.3   *Example screenshots from gaze data collected in Sobuh's study [36]
showing visual attention (directed towards the hand and 'GCA') while
approaching and grasping the carton. Gaze is seen to fixate on the
glass during pouring*

et al. [37] studied gaze behaviour while lifting an object and placing it into a cylinder. In addition, real-world usage was measured by wrist-worn activity monitors over a period of 7 days. Surprisingly, real-world usage did not correlate with measures of gaze behaviour, even in this larger sample. Hebert *et al.* [41] compared visuomotor performance of 8 prosthesis users and 16 controls across 2 tasks, 1 conducted in front of the participant and for which over compression would result in spillage, and another in which the task required a trunk movement and placement of object at different heights. They found different visuomotor performance across the two tasks, suggesting prosthesis users may employ different visual strategies depending on the objects and their locations relative to the body. The combined results of these studies clearly demonstrate a disruption to visual strategies of movement control upon use of a prosthesis. However, the lack of clear training or expertise effects raises questions over whether models of 'expert' gaze derived from literature on healthy limb use provide an appropriate benchmark for comparison with prosthesis users.

Laboratory studies using eye-tracking have focused predominantly on tasks performed with a single limb (an exception is in Bouwsema *et al.* [13], who included a condition which involved hand-to-hand transfer). In contrast, Raveh *et al.* [42] used eye-tracking as a way of assessing attentional demands during dual-task performance in 12 myoelectric users. The dual-task set-up involved moving a car on a computer screen with the user's healthy limb, while simultaneously performing a variety of real-world grasp and manipulation tasks with their prosthesis. Vibrotactile stimulation was provided during object contact in half the trials and was predicted to help object manipulation by providing sensory information about contact with the object. Gaze was measured to the screen task rather than to the grasping task and used as an index of how much the vibrotactile feedback freed up attention from the prosthesis. When feedback was present, there were generally fewer gaze shifts between screen and limb and more time spent attending to the screen, although neither of these trends reached .05 level of significance. Although the screen-based task here is somewhat artificial, the strength of studies which involve both limbs is that they begin to shed light on the complex nature of bilateral movements that make up many real-world actions (see [43]).

3.3.2   Kinematics

Although there has been some work on the kinetics of the upper limb, there has been little or no work published on the use of inverse or forward dynamics models to evaluate prostheses. Therefore, this section focuses on the application of techniques to measure kinematics. Kinematics is a branch of dynamics that deals with motion alone.

Motion analysis began with the measurement of human walking (gait). This is a simple, well-recognised activity that is broadly the same for all people but significant deviations from this 'norm' can reflect problems with joint and body segment biomechanics or neural control. Analysis consists of recording the motion and then transforming the data to match a single stride, from heel strike (when the foot first contacts with the ground) through all of the stance phases to toe off, when the foot leaves the ground, and then finishing after the swing phase with the next heel strike. When transformed into percentage of the stride, the data is very comparable and differences may be both relatively easy to identify and relate to deviations from normal control and mechanics. It is a standard tool for analysis, treatment planning and tracking in many areas of physical medicine.

However, in general, upper limb movements are much less constrained and perhaps partly as a result there are considerably fewer publications on upper limb kinematics than on gait. Nevertheless, techniques originally developed for gait analysis have been applied to the analysis of upper limb movement and for the evaluation of upper limb prostheses. This section will introduce measurement methods then review the characteristic changes to kinematics seen during the performance of goal-directed tasks, including structured task sets such as SHAP and B&B.

3.3.2.1 Measurement techniques

Full motion analysis requires each body segment to be recorded with the six degrees of freedom (three translational and three rotational). There are a range of techniques used to measure upper limb motion, ranging from markerless tracking in which the basic kinematic form of the limb is assumed and what is viewed is warped to fit the motion [44], approaches based on wearable (typically inertial-magnetic) sensors [45], to the methods traditionally used in gait analysis, stereophotogrammetry.

Markerless motion tracking is used in common consumer-based motion tracking products, such as (the no longer supported) Kinect system and Leap motion. The Kinect system is sufficiently flexible that a person with an upper limb absence can play in the same game with anatomically intact players without undue disadvantage. The image of the body is simply distorted so, for example for a person with a transradial absence, the short arm pushes the centre of the body towards the intact arm. However, its use in research is limited, because the approximations involved in fitting the model to the observed data mean that accuracy is limited. Other issues include sensitivity to lighting conditions, which can lead to tracking problems [46]. Inertial-magnetic sensors (often called magnetic-inertial measurement units or MIMUs) typically include a 3-axis accelerometer (essentially a mass on springs, the movement of which can be used to infer the inertial forces acting on the mass and gravity), 3-axis rate gyroscope (which measures angular velocity) and a magnetometer (which measures the orientation of the sensor with respect to the Earth's magnetic field). Sophisticated methods, such as Kalman filter state estimation, are used to integrate the data from the sensors to give an estimate of the orientation of the sensor with respect to a reference frame defined by the Earth's magnetic field and gravity [47]. By aligning the coordinate frames of sensors on adjoining segments with anatomical features (either through careful placement or performance of well-defined movements to identify joint rotation axes) [45], joint angle trajectories and associated derivatives can be obtained.

Stereophotogrammetry is a technique which uses infrared cameras to track the location of reflective markers in a calibrated space. In order to define the 3D position and 3D orientation of an object (in this case a body segment) in space, a minimum of three markers are needed to establish a coordinate frame. There are standard approaches to the mapping of the cluster-based coordinate frames into more meaningful upper limb coordinate systems [48,49]. These approaches can be used to estimate, from marker data on adjoining segments, parameters such as joint angle trajectories and their rate of change (angular velocities). Marker data also obviously gives the location of the segment of interest in space and associated data on linear translation, velocity and accelerations. The drawback of the marker-based kinematic tracking is the amount of time required to set up a subject and process the resulting data. The result is that the numbers recorded in experiments relying on optical tracking are usually limited and analysis is generally complex.

Finally, and somewhat separately, as powered prostheses often include sensors on device configuration (e.g. hand pose), the kinematics of the prosthesis itself could be obtained from this. A few recent studies have reported logged data on grasp usage as an outcome measure [50]. A more in-depth discussion of the value of real-world measures such as these is given later in this chapter.

3.3.2.2   Goal-directed movement in anatomically intact participants

To interpret kinematics-based observations of behaviours in upper limb prosthesis users, it is useful to understand the basic characteristics of upper limb behaviours in anatomically intact, healthy participants.

A useful framework for considering upper limb motor control in general was proposed by Bernstein (see [24] for a good overview of the concept in the context of prosthetics). Bongers quoted Bernstein's definition of dexterity as follows: 'Dexterity is the ability to find a motor solution for any external situation, that is, to adequately solve any emerging motor problem correctly (i.e. adequately and accurately), quickly (with respect to both decision making and achieving a correct result), rationally (i.e. expediently and economically), and resourcefully (i.e. quick-wittedly and initiatively)'. This definition raises several key concepts which will be explored in the following sections. For example, the major joints of the upper limb form a kinematically redundant system. As an example, consider holding a cup with your elbow in a moderately flexed posture on the table; while not moving your hand or the cup, your arm can be rotated about the long axis connecting the shoulder joint and wrist. This illustrates that there is more than one solution to the set of joint angles which position and orient your hand in such a way as to hold the cup on the table. This redundancy means that during a reach-to-grasp movement the human motor control system is continuously solving the complex (inverse) kinematic problem of accurately, quickly and economically moving the hand towards a suitable grasp on the object. Second, the human motor system solves this problem in a highly (cognitively) efficient manner, based on muscle synergies which form the building blocks for goal-directed movement. As discussed earlier, visual attention during reach-to-grasp is used largely for planning actions and, as will be discussed later, requires little cognitive resources. As an example, think about reaching for a cup of tea while talking to a friend. The conversation can continue uninterrupted by the demands of reaching for and acquiring the object. Reflecting on the immensely complex problems of dynamically configuring the joints of the upper limb while also stabilising the trunk to position the appropriately configured hand around the cup handle highlights the remarkable sophistication of the human motor control system.

Common paradigms used to characterise upper limb behaviours in anatomically intact participants have been the goal-directed movements, such as pointing and reaching to grasp objects, typically measured under laboratory conditions.

The kinematics of the arm and hand during reach-to-grasp movements have been widely studied. Jeannerod in the 1980s studying reaching to grasp cylindrical objects proposed that there were two components to the movement [51]. The hand transport component, during which the hand is moved towards the object, and the grasp component, during which the hand and finger posture is prepared, based on the object properties. Stereotypical behaviours are observed in each of these phases. For example, hand aperture increases smoothly until it reaches its peak around 70% of the time needed to reach the object then starts to close as it approaches the object. The hand aperture is coupled to object size and wrist velocity during reach is characterised by bell-shaped curves, which scale with distance. A more in-depth overview of upper limb kinematics during a reach-to-grasp movement is given in [52].

3.3.2.3 Kinematics of goal-directed movement in prosthesis users

Some of the first studies comparing the trajectory of the arm and hand during the performance of tasks by participants with limb absence were reported in the early 1980s by Fraser and Wing [53,54]. With a view to informing the development of training methods, they reported a case study of a participant with left-sided congenital limb absence below the elbow. They used early motion analysis equipment to compare her performance on a simple reach-to-grasp task, using her voluntary-opening body-powered prosthetic hand, with her performance with her (right) anatomical hand. The subject was slower when performing the task using her prosthesis, and unlike the anatomical hand showed a plateau in the hand aperture-time trajectory, reflecting *normal* hand–arm coordination early in reach-to-grasp but delayed onset of hand closure on the object.

This series of papers was followed by a rather extended period during which there was relatively little attention paid to the kinematics of upper limb prosthetic users. Notable contributions over this period included work by Hogan's group at MIT, evaluating the performance of amputees when carrying out constrained tasks, including crank turning [55], pointing and tracking (at different frequencies) [56]. The Doeringer study involved six unilateral above-elbow users of body-powered prostheses and compared performance using the intact limb with the prosthetic limb. In a pointing task, the more experienced users were able to position their body-powered end effectors to a similar degree of accuracy to their intact limb. However, performance with the body-powered end effector was significantly worse on a dynamic tracking task. They also observed a greater number of peaks in the end effector velocity profiles seen during a dynamic tracking task than was the case for the intact limb.

Although there followed a few 'observational' studies of kinematics measured during the performance of ADLs (e.g. [57,58]), the decade since 2010 has seen a renewed interest in the field.

A series of studies by the Bongers group led the way in this area [13,59–62]. The studies were grounded in human motor control and motor learning theory and addressed both body-powered and myoelectric prostheses. In summary, prehension in both users of myoelectric and body-powered prostheses is slower and shows a relatively long deceleration phase at the end of the reach phase; the start of reaching does not necessarily coincide with the start of grasping (aperture change), nor do the end points coincide; and the aperture profile shows a clear plateau [24].

3.3.2.4   Motion capture combined with existing tests

The majority of studies have tended to focus either on highly constrained tasks (typically reaching for and grasping a small number of regular-shaped objects) [13], or on the performance of ADLs, such as drinking from a cup [58].

A small number of studies have explored kinematic analysis of the performance of a traditional clinical outcome measure. Kyberd *et al.* have shown the potential merits of studying upper limb kinematics during the performance of the SHAP [63] (see Section 3.2.3). The way in which SHAP is designed means that the object locations relative to the desk on which the test is performed is fixed, and the user has to return their hand to the start posture (on top of the timing button) before the subsequent activity attempt. While such constraints may not be unique to SHAP, Kyberd *et al.* recognised that the constrained environment lends itself to applying a linear scaling to the kinematic data similar to gait. In this instance, one 'cycle' is defined as starting when the button is pressed to turn the timer on, and ending when the button is pressed again, turning it off. Other clinical tests have also been combined with motion capture. For instance, the Alberta-based BLINC lab team have used kinematic analysis during the performance of the box and block test [64] also worth noting that groups are beginning to explore combining standard clinical tests with other outcome measures, such as gaze behaviour and electroencephalography (EEG) (covered in the next section).

3.3.2.5   Kinematic variability

Anatomically intact upper limb movement during the performance of goal-directed movement is generally rather smooth and follows rather characteristic trajectories. However, when learning to use a tool, people typically show a high degree of variability in their kinematics in the early stages of learning, which reduces with practice. Indeed, some have argued that a reduction in the variability of movement (at a given speed) is a core feature of skill learning [65].

A prosthesis user has by definition a reduced set of proprioceptive information, is generally more reliant on vision for control and, in the case of myoelectric prosthesis users, has to deal with a degree of both delay and uncertainty in the intention–action chain. These factors may also contribute to the observed behaviours that have been reported in two studies, which used different approaches to characterising movement variability.

Major *et al.* 2014 characterised joint angle trajectory variability in six able-bodied controls and seven myoelectric transradial prosthesis users during the performance of goal-directed tasks taken from the SHAP outcome measure [66]. Joint angle trajectories at the shoulder and elbow were calculated and the variability of these parameters over five repeats of each task were calculated using two approaches. First, the standard deviation of each degree of freedom time trajectory (defined in the paper to be a measure of absolute kinematic variability), and second, the adjusted coefficient of multiple determination, a measure which reflects the similarity of curves (defined to be a measure of repeatability). The authors found that absolute kinematic variability was greater for prosthesis users for all degrees of freedom in each task, although this was only significant for the degrees of freedom which showed greater range of motion. They also found that repeatability was strongly associated with 'prosthesis experience'. A subsequent study by Thies *et al.* 2017 characterised variability [67] based on the motion of a body segment, in this case the forearm, rather than joint angle trajectories. This study simulated the outputs of a wrist-worn accelerometer during the performance of goal-directed activities and characterised the trial–trial variability of the trajectories using a dynamic time-warping approach [68]. This approach allows for the separation of a measure of timing variability from trajectory variability and the study found that the timing variability was greater in amputee users of myoelectric prostheses than in anatomically intact controls, and in anatomically intact participants learning to use a myoelectric prosthesis simulator, timing variability decreased with practice. These two studies support further investigation of movement variability as an outcome measure.

3.3.2.6 Workspace

A body-powered prosthesis is controlled via an operating cable, typically a Bowden cable, which runs from a shoulder-worn or torso-worn harness through to the active TD, usually a split hook or a mechanical hand. Shoulder or upper arm movement, normally bi-scapula abduction and/or humeral flexion, applies tension through the harness and the attached operating cable, which, in turn, can open or close the TD, thereby enabling the user to grasp and hold objects. However, as the cable does not pass through the prosthesis joint centres, the path length between the harness and the TD is posture dependent. Setting up a body-powered prosthesis requires a compromise length of cable to be determined; too long and the shoulder range of movement may be insufficient to take up the cable slack in some postures, meaning the user will not be able to operate the end effector; too short and the reachable workspace will be limited by this. Building on techniques used to assess workspace in other populations [69] has used kinematic analysis techniques to study this problem [70]. Such an approach would also be interesting to apply to other types of upper limb prosthesis, where function may be somewhat posture dependent [37,71].

3.3.2.7 Other approaches (gesture intensity/frequency)

Finally, as the upper limb is not only used for functional purposes but also as a means of communicating, a recent study by Maimon-Mor [72] has captured the frequency with which upper limb amputees gesture. They proposed that the use of a prosthesis to gesture as a means of communication may be reflective of the degree of embodiment of the prosthesis. The authors invited participants to describe a video and a number of objects, designed to encourage gesturing. The frequency and magnitude of gestures were captured using video and wrist-worn accelerometers, respectively. They found that both amputees and people with unilateral congenital limb absence used their prosthesis to gesture but differed to anatomically intact controls in the degree of reliance on the other (intact/dominant) hand. Interestingly, the degree of reliance on the intact hand in gestures correlated with a measure of upper limb activity of the prosthesis in everyday life.

3.3.3 Eye-tracking and EEG

EEG records the brain's electrical activity from electrodes placed on the scalp. EEG can detect a range of cortical waveforms which are used to infer levels of mental activity (e.g. sleep through to wakefulness to high levels of mental effort) across different sites of the cortex. EEG data can be captured with high spatial resolution, providing insight into the level of cognitive effort required from tasks on an ongoing basis. One type of neural activity, the alpha wave, is associated with skilled performance through its inhibitory role in cortical activation, whereby higher alpha power corresponds to less cortical activity, which is an indication of a reduction in cognitive effort. This principle has been applied by Parr *et al.* [40] to investigate the level of cognitive effort involved in prosthesis use and to validate findings from eye-tracking. In their study, 20 able-bodied participants performed a jar-lifting task (taken from the SHAP) with both the anatomical hand and while wearing a prosthesis simulator. Consistent with earlier studies, gaze was directed more often at the prosthetic hand than at the anatomical hand, indicating an increased reliance on vision when using the prosthesis simulator. The EEG results demonstrated that lower global alpha level, indicating higher cortical activity, was involved in controlling the prosthesis simulator. The authors interpreted the combined eye-tracking and EEG results as showing increased cognitive effort and reliance on vision when first learning to control a prosthetic device.

Another potential value of EEG is in elucidating the coordination of different cognitive and motor processes which support ongoing movement and how these change over time. Such insight is valuable for evaluating the effectiveness of different training regimes. 'Alpha connectivity' refers to synchrony in the alpha signal between two brain areas, reflecting high functional connectivity between those areas [40]. Expertise is reflected in a reduction of connectivity between motor planning areas of the brain, and those involved in verbal–analytical processes. Verbal–analytical involvement suggests conscious control of action, reflective of early stages in motor learning [40]. In their second experiment, Parr *et al.* compared two training techniques, one where novice prosthesis simulator users were required to explicitly focus on their movements (movement training), and a second on which the users focused on imitating the pattern of gaze employed by an expert (gaze training; GT). GT is intended to expedite learning to a more advanced, implicit form of motor control. Indeed, their study demonstrated greater improvement in task performance following GT, and this was reflected in reduced alpha connectivity between motor planning and verbal–analytical brain regions [40]. While questions remain about what constitutes an expert pattern of gaze for prosthesis users, the results from Parr *et al.* provide a compelling example of how EEG allows insight into mechanisms behind prosthesis learning that are not accessible through observational or self-report measures.

3.3.4 Discussion

Laboratory-based outcome measures have developed rapidly over the last 10–15 years, with the emergence of entirely new areas (e.g. gaze behaviours and EEG analysis) and significant growth in approaches to kinematic analysis. Gaze behaviour analysis is at an early stage in its development, although already having established some key issues. For example, consistent across multiple studies is the finding that patterns of gaze behaviours in users of myoelectric prostheses differ markedly from those seen in anatomically intact participants. However, recent work suggesting prosthesis users may employ different visual strategies depending on the objects and their locations relative to the body [41] raises questions about whether the gaze-based metrics of skilled behaviour derived from studies of tool use are directly transferable to prosthesis users.

Studies of kinematics of prosthesis users have established some key issues. For example, transradial users of both body-powered and myoelectric prostheses show characteristic patterns in both the reach and grasping phases when moving to acquire an object. A small number of studies have begun to reveal the changes to these behaviours over practice, and these observations may help to inform the reader on the choice of parameters reflective of skill. Other metrics which appear to be associated with experience (and may change in a predictable way with practice) include variability of both joint and segment trajectories during the performance of goal-directed actions. It is interesting to note that wearable-based approaches are starting to emerge and studies of less constrained movements, such as gestures, have shown early promise. Finally, an adjunct to gaze behaviours, EEG is beginning to be explored.

3.4 Real-world techniques

In the previous sections, we have considered several methods to evaluate how well a person is able to use their prosthesis; however, the conclusive test of the value of an upper limb prosthesis is not the person's ability to use it, but how often and when they choose to wear it, and how and when they use it, in their everyday lives. Various surveys have suggested that perhaps between 20% and 40% of upper limb prostheses are *rejected** by their users, depending on the type of prosthesis and the age group of the users surveyed. Clearly, however, well those who report rejecting their prosthesis can perform tasks with their prosthesis, the value of their prosthesis is outweighed by other negative factors. Further, if the prehensile function of a prosthesis is rarely used in everyday life, then it is difficult to properly interpret the results of the many outcome measures which primarily focus on assessing the prehensile function. Indeed, as discussed earlier, the recognition that people with limb loss will find their own way of achieving upper limb tasks, which may or may not fully exploit the prehensile functions of the prosthesis, underlies some of the more sophisticated clinical measures, such as the ACMC [7]. However, measures such as the ACMC are

---

*The term device rejection is not consistently defined in the literature. Consequently, determining the level of rejection and comparing results is difficult and this may partly explain the high variation seen in reported rejection rates.

time-consuming and difficult to carry out, requiring skilled assessors; more importantly, all observational outcome measures are inherently limited in terms of where and how they are carried out. These tests at best provide a snapshot of behaviours, under observation for a very short period of time (a few hours at most). How well such behaviours reflect overall real-world behaviours is unknown and, until recently this has not been measurable in an objective manner.

For many years, the primary methods of determining how much a prosthesis was worn and used was by user self-report and/or visual inspection of the prosthesis for signs of wear-and-tear. Although such approaches offer some insight, they are inherently subjective. Self-report is known to be liable to bias and recall errors [73]; equally importantly, the questions posed often only consider average prosthesis wear time and therefore do not consider variations in the patterns of prosthesis wear over time [74].

By adding sensors to the prosthesis that record movement, or using other instrumentation, we can objectively assess clinically meaningful outcomes relating to aspects of prosthesis wear/use over prolonged periods of home use. In addition, in the case of people with unilateral absence, there is an opportunity to compare the activity of the prosthetic and anatomic limbs. In this section, we introduce the latest techniques and findings in a new but rapidly growing field.

3.4.1   Real-world monitoring

The value of non-invasive, wearable sensors to rehabilitation practice are widely reported [75–78], predominantly in the assessment of walking [75]. By placing movement sensors on the upper limbs and/or torso, it is now possible to gather high-quality data on upper limb behaviours in the real world [75].

Typically, inertial sensors are used to measure upper limb movement, although other approaches have been tried. Some of the early incarnations of activity monitoring for the upper limb were included by Vega-Gonzalez and Granat [79], who used an arm-mounted, fluid-filled tube attached to a pressure transducer, which gave a continuous output proportional to the vertical distance between the wrist (location of end of tube) and the shoulder (location of the transducer). Nevertheless, by far the most common of the inertial sensors used in upper limb activity monitoring has been the accelerometer. An accelerometer uses a mass on a suspension, the movement of which is dependent on the gravitational and inertial forces acting on it. In situations where the device is static, the only force acting on the mass is gravity and hence it is possible to estimate the orientation of the accelerometer reference frame relative to vertical. In cases where the device is moving in a general way, the interpretation of the accelerometer outputs is more complex. Commercial systems incorporating 3-axis accelerometers are available from several companies, including ActiGraph, ActivInsights and Axivity. These wrist-worn sensors may also include GPS, light sensors and pulse monitors, the latter can be used (in anatomically intact participants to infer whether or not the monitors are being worn). Typically, the output of accelerometers is made available to the user either in the form of 'raw' acceleration values, or 'activity counts'. The algorithms that use acceleration data to calculate activity counts are generally proprietary software, but a general overview is given in [80]. An example of an algorithm to estimate activity counts is given in [81]. At present, off-the-shelf systems do not offer validated algorithms specifically for the analysis of upper limb actions [75]; however, algorithms using one or two wrist-worn sensors to assess upper limb symmetry based on activity counts have been published, as well as some algorithms for the classification of simple activities [74,82–86]. The most common approaches are reviewed next.

3.4.2   Real-world assessment of upper limb activity

Most commonly real-world upper limb activity has been analysed using accelerometers, with metrics based on the magnitude and/or duration of arm movements [87]. In order to understand the impact of a unilateral upper limb impairment, two sensors are generally worn (one on each limb) in order to measure the activity of both the impaired and unimpaired limbs. The movement of the impaired limb can then be referenced to the movement of the unimpaired limb. In this way, it has been possible to differentiate people who have experienced a stroke from healthy participants with no neurological impairments [83,88]. Levels of activity seen in the dominant and non-dominant limb in unimpaired young participants have been shown to be quite evenly balanced, a finding which is consistent across studies [87].

Accelerometers have been widely used for the assessment of lower limb prosthesis wear/use (in particular ambulatory measures), but only recently have they been considered for use as an outcome measure in upper limb prosthetics. In a study by Makin *et al.* [82], accelerometers were used to validate a questionnaire on limb usage strategies. One sensor was placed on the wrist of the anatomically intact arm, and a second was worn on the proximal aspect of the affected upper arm. Based on a thresholding algorithm, the number of discrete movements of each arm was calculated. A laterality ratio, defined as the difference between the number of movements recorded on each limb, divided by the sum of movements on each limb was calculated. The laterality ratio reflected the frequency with which users moved their residual limb relative to their intact limb. Due to the placement of the sensors, this data did not inform on prosthesis wear or use, but more broadly on the use of the affected limb versus the anatomically intact limb. In a study undertaken by Chadwell *et al.*, participants wore sensors on both wrists (anatomically intact and prosthetic) [38]. In their subsequent work, Chadwell *et al.* published algorithms for the removal of prosthesis non-wear periods [89] and novel methods for the visualisation of prosthesis use [74]. Finally, Lang *et al.* who have developed a range of methods for the assessment of upper limb symmetry for use in stroke rehabilitation showed that their methods can also be used with data from a prosthesis user [88].

In the following sections, the algorithms that have used inertial measurement units (IMUs) to estimate when the sensors (and prosthesis) are worn, and the metrics on prosthesis usage, are reviewed.

3.4.2.1   Non-wear algorithms

There is no gold standard with respect to recording sensor (and prosthesis) wear times. Activity monitors offer the potential to develop objective measures of wear; however, the non-wear algorithms developed for these sensors have generally been developed for hip-worn sensors, and most have not been validated in a home setting.

Self-reported wear/non-wear would be expected to be the gold standard; however, participants often vary significantly in the accuracy of self-reported wear times. One of the most common monitor suppliers, ActiGraph [90], offers two non-wear algorithms ('Troiano 2007' and 'Choi 2011'); however, these were both developed based on data from hip-worn monitors. A recent study by Knaier *et al.* [91] aimed to validate these automated non-wear algorithms for detection of non-wear of wrist-worn sensors. The study showed the Choi algorithm [92] to demonstrate the greatest agreement with self-reported wear times; however, this algorithm is unable to detect periods of non-wear lasting less than 90 min. It should be noted that a prosthesis may be removed for shorter periods than 90 min, thus reducing the accuracy of this algorithm for the detection of non-wear in this cohort. The same study [91] highlighted that reducing the minimum non-wear period from 90 min would reduce the risk of overestimating the wear time (by reducing Type II errors); however, the number of Type I errors (inaccurately stating the sensor was not worn) occurring during sleep may increase. As very few (or no) people wear a prosthesis during sleep, for the purpose of improving the accuracy of detecting prosthesis non-wear, reduction of the minimum non-wear period would be recommended. Chadwell *et al.* developed a method to detect prosthesis non-wear periods which involved a shorter threshold [37,89]. Chadwell's methods were more complex, allowing for some small isolated spikes of low-level activity to occur (<15 counts) during a non-wear period to avoid misclassification. The threshold for wear/non-wear was based around a 20-min period of consecutive activity/inactivity; for more details on the identification of a transition between wear/non-wear, see [37,88]. It is worth noting that there are some features which these non-wear algorithms are unable to account for. For example, Figure 3.4 shows a comparison between the calculated and self-reported prosthesis wear over a single day. In this example there are two portions of misclassified data (highlighted by the arrows). During these periods the participant was travelling in a vehicle but was not wearing the prosthesis. The vibrations of the vehicle appeared to the algorithm as prosthesis wear. The extraction of wear (both sensor wear and prosthesis wear), and meaningful movement data from a recorded data set requires further work. Interestingly, if we could detect the person walking [93], we could improve our understanding of meaningful movements by isolating movements due to arm swing during walking. It should however be noted that swinging the arm during gait is still an important measure with respect to the prosthesis and as such could be categorised as a separate upper limb activity; arm swing on the affected side demonstrates that the person is not rigidly holding the arm still during natural movements.

3.4.2.2   Metrics to capture prosthesis use

It is important that we differentiate prosthesis wear from prosthesis use as they measure distinctly different things. Research has shown that some prosthesis wearers may still be heavily reliant on the anatomically intact arm during periods when the prosthesis is worn. Metrics to evaluate prosthesis (and/or residual limb) use to date have included the following:

* **Magnitude ratio** [88]: The magnitude ratio is a natural log of the vector magnitude of the activity counts from the prosthesis-located sensor divided by the vector

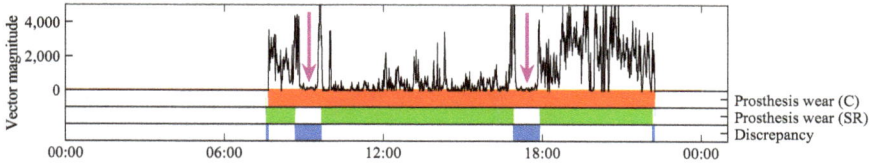

Figure 3.4   *Vector magnitude of tri-axial activity counts recorded from a prosthesis worn ActiGraph over a 24-h period. Adapted from the supplementary material of Chadwell et al. [37]. In red are the periods labelled as prosthesis wear by the non-wear algorithm (C), and in green is the self-reported (SR) wear. In blue is the discrepancy. Two periods marked by arrows were incorrectly identified as wear by Chadwell's non-wear algorithm. During these periods the participant reported to have removed their prosthesis to drive*

magnitude of the activity counts from the sensor on the anatomically intact arm. Filtered accelerometer data from the anatomical and prosthetic limb sensors, sampled at 1 Hz, were first converted to activity counts. The activity count values from the sensor on the prosthetic arm were divided by the activity count from the sensor on the intact limb and transformed using the natural log. To account for periods when the activity count on either limb was zero, a magnitude ratio of +7 was assigned to periods of unilateral prosthesis use, and −7 for periods of unilateral intact arm use. This rather unusual approach to the analysis makes it quite difficult to interpret the results.

- **Laterality ratio** [82]: This measure was used for assessment of the residual limb use, not prosthesis use; hence, the different terminology used. The number of movements of each limb is calculated, and a ratio is given based on the number of movements made by the anatomically intact limb minus the number of movements on the affected side, divided by the total number of movements across both limbs. A movement event was defined by an observed change in the magnitude of measured acceleration within a specified time window exceeding a threshold value, conditional on the event being preceded and followed by a period of no movement.

- **Percentage reliance on the anatomically intact arm** [74]: This was calculated by dividing the vector magnitude of the activity counts recorded from the sensors on the dominant/anatomical arm by the total vector magnitude across both arms. Any data points where the vector magnitude on each sensor was zero were removed from the analysis.

- **Unilateral ratio** [74]: This is the ratio between the total duration of unilateral prosthesis use and total duration of unilateral use of the anatomically intact arm.

- **Bilateral magnitude** [88]: This is the sum of the vector magnitude of both arms.

It is worth pointing out that all these methods are based on data from wrist-mounted accelerometers. This obviously provides no information on whether or not the prehension function is being used. As discussed later in this chapter, some multi-articulating myoelectric prostheses log this data, but as yet the authors are unaware of any publications which have integrated these data with the data from activity monitoring sensors.

3.4.3   Discussion

Wearable sensors allow us to quickly, cheaply and easily measure, currently rather crude but informative, important aspects of use and wear in everyday life. It is worth noting that a recent study in upper limb myoelectric users showed no correlation between metrics reflecting the balance of activity between the intact and prosthetic limbs, and measures of performance taken in the lab [37]. This suggests that activity monitoring could be used to complement other approaches.

Although there are a number of studies highlighting the benefits of activity monitors for the assessment of real-world upper limb activity [87,94], they are not without their limitations. The data loggers within off-the-shelf activity monitoring sensors are known to be affected by clock drift [95,96] which introduces problems when combining data from two sensors. Further, the field is still in its infancy and key questions remain, including the optimal epoch length used in the estimation of activity counts; a recent study showed differences in outcomes with different epoch lengths [97]. For an overview of activity monitoring in prosthetics, the reader is referred to Chadwell's recent review paper [98].

Currently the measures presented here do not allow us to distinguish specific movements, or to evaluate the quality of movements, although these are areas which are being developed. For example, a recent study using a head-mounted camera showed promise in revealing detail on the nature of prosthesis use in a home setting [43]. However, the analysis of these data is currently a very time-consuming process, making its routine use impractical for the time being. Of potentially more relevance is the analysis of data logged from the prosthesis itself. Multi-articulating myoelectric prostheses may be logging the number of times each grip pattern has been used, and how often the motors have been activated, and a recent publication reported these data [50]. The potential to exploit this development will be discussed in more detail in the following section.

In the future, we should be looking to monitor movements of the intact limb, activations of the TD and any other components such as a wrist or an elbow (including details of the type/speed/extent of movement), and exploit parameters such as pressure or lux inside the socket to help one to determine whether the prosthesis was worn. Additionally, if activity monitors could also be placed on the residual limb, we could better understand how limb use differs when the prosthesis is/is not worn. However, it is important to consider that increasing the number of sensors can negatively impact compliance. Thus, in future it could be useful to integrate as many of the sensors as possible into the limb itself, while also considering the effect this may have on prosthesis weight [99]. If users were able to upload their own data remotely via Bluetooth, this could increase the potential benefits of these low-contact methods clinically over the longer term (e.g. if wear or use appears to drop, the user could be automatically notified, and it could be suggested that they may need to visit the clinic).

Such approaches require further usability investigations and careful addressing of privacy issues before going ahead. Some of these issues are discussed next.

3.5 Data science, big data, standards and the future

The massive increase in easily accessible, structured, fine-grained data on human behaviours in the real world, combined with new approaches to data analytics, opens up opportunities to address health-related questions on a scale, and in ways which were simply not available in previous decades. Before going on to discuss these, it is worth reflecting on the limitations imposed by our current approaches to clinical evaluation.

3.5.1 Small-scale, short-term studies

In contrast to the mainstream medical literature, where large, randomised, controlled trials are common, the studies in upper limb prosthetics are much smaller in scale. This is due in part to the small and geographically widely distributed nature of the populations (at least in the European Union (EU) and North America, where the vast majority of such studies have taken place). Further, with a few exceptions, the majority of studies in upper limb prosthetics have not attempted long term following of participants. This is a major failing; in contrast to acute medicine, for example prosthetics rehabilitation is a long-term process often requiring frequent modifications to both the socket and prosthesis hardware and prescription. However, current studies are generally failing to capture data over sufficient time to reflect this clinical and user reality. Again, logistics make such studies difficult and particularly so in the small cohorts available to participate in any given centre in which even small numbers of dropouts could mean the trial having to terminate. Finally, a large proportion of studies in the upper limb prosthetics area recruit anatomically intact participants, making clinical inferences from the results very difficult.

3.5.2 Study bias

The way in which studies are currently designed means that they are expensive to run, require highly trained staff typically at the sites where data collection takes place and require participants to travel for data collection. Unsurprisingly, the vast majority take place in North America and the EU. By contrast, the majority of people with upper limb absence live in lower- and middle-income countries and hence do not get enrolled in clinical studies. This means that the results of clinical evaluations are inherently biased towards populations representative of the richer nations.

3.5.3 Absence of useful data on prostheses characteristics and lack of standardisation on participant characteristics

With a few notable exceptions [38,39], the description of the prosthesis being evaluated is either absent or very limited in detail and in many cases simply reports the trade name of the device. Studies in which the prosthesis being assessed are described only in terms of a trade name quickly become out of date (when a new version of the product is launched). Further, without some kind of model to represent the important properties of the prosthesis, it is difficult to unpick why one is better than another. In this respect, the lower limb prosthetics design community is somewhat more advanced than the corresponding upper limb community [100].

Although participant demographics are reported, such as age, level of limb absence, whether limb absence is from birth or acquired, there is no commonly adopted standard on what details should be reported.

3.5.4   *Limited adoption of standard approaches to measuring outcomes*

Although there are a number of review articles that have attempted to identify the set of (clinical) outcome measures which should be used in evaluation [3,4], the recommendations still leave researchers with a wide range of options. Further, none of the recent reviews cover outcome measures based on kinematics or real-world monitoring. These factors combine to make reuse of the data for secondary analysis, for example meta-analysis, very difficult. With one or two recent exceptions [89,101], open data has yet to have a significant impact on the field.

3.5.5   *Data science and big data*

The move towards real-world measures opens up opportunities to address the limitations with current approaches discussed earlier. Such real-world approaches to capturing and analysing data at scale are rapidly gaining traction in other domains [102], and this section will introduce some of the key concepts and then discuss how they may be applied in upper limb prosthetics.

The US National Institute for Health defines data science as an 'interdisciplinary field of inquiry in which quantitative and analytical approaches, processes, and systems are developed and used to extract knowledge and insights from increasingly large and/or complex sets of data' [103]. Data science researchers refer to large data and big data and the distinction between the two is based not only on the size of the data set but also on the analysis methods adopted.

There are already studies which exploit data from wearables and fitness apps to explore research questions in public health [104]. For example, a recent study used a smartphone-based app and the in-built IMUs to log step counts from over 700,000 users in order to identify the relationships between walking intensity and obesity. The UK Biobank initiative is another example of where data sets have been collected to address health research questions at scale.

Upper limb prosthetics is a field which could benefit significantly from such new approaches. At its most basic, consider the issue of how often people use their devices and in which context. Such questions are common to many of the questionnaires used in clinical studies, suggesting they are important issues. As pointed out earlier, we currently largely rely on self-report to capture these data, which provide at best a heavily summarised description with significant potential for bias and recall errors. It is widely believed that the more advanced prosthetic devices log data on use of their devices, although the authors are only aware of one study [50] which has reported such data. If these data could be combined with data from, for example a consumer product such as Google Maps, which can track the location of the user over time, our knowledge of prosthesis use and context could increase dramatically.

More exciting is the prospect of using similar methods to gain a much better insight into the characteristics which make a prosthesis of value to the user. For example, we know from various surveys that users do not like the weight of current prostheses, want more controllable degrees of freedom and improved reliability. However, such descriptive statements are of limited value to designers, who need to understand, for example the weightings of these factors, how they vary between users (is there a need for bespoke elements to devices), and importantly, whether a new design which attempts to address one or more of these issues is better than previous. If the community could move towards engineering standards with which to characterise the functional properties of prostheses, this opens up the opportunities for large-scale, real-world studies which explore the relationships between well-defined models of prostheses and real-world use. Such a framework would be challenging to set up but could lead to a transformation in the field. A small number of studies have explored the characterisation of upper limb prostheses. For example, Smit [105] used a simple model of mechanical work done during opening and closing to characterise the mechanical efficiency of these devices and Chadwell *et al.* [38] characterised myoelectric single degree of freedom devices in terms of the delay from EMG onset of aperture movement. A first attempt to explore how device (interface and user) characteristics correlate with actual use has been reported in [37], but there is considerable scope for further work in the area.

There are clearly many obstacles to be overcome before the approaches discussed in this section can become widespread. For example, they would rely on partnerships between prosthetic companies, academic researchers and other companies or organisations from outside the prosthetics field. Although there are some examples of partnerships between researchers and prosthetics companies, these are relatively few in number and the authors are unaware of any partnerships with consumer app-type companies to address such questions. All of the previous approaches rely on sensible approaches to data protection and other ethical issues. The discussion of these issues lies outside of the scope of this chapter, but the reader is referred to [104] for a good overview.

3.6 Discussion and conclusions

Although not comprehensive, the chapter has hopefully provided the reader with an overview of the main approaches available to the evaluation of upper limb prostheses, which may help when deciding how to address a particular evaluation problem.

This chapter began with a discussion of the problems inherent to the evaluation of upper limb prostheses. Central to this is the fact that we use our upper limb(s) for a very wide range of operations, for a wide range of purposes. This means that any single outcome measure is unlikely to capture the full value of a prosthesis to the person.

Nevertheless, the so-called 'traditional approaches' to evaluation can provide easy to understand data on a person's ability to perform activities with their prosthesis. Commonly used approaches include the ACMC [7] and the SHAP test [10], two measures which take perhaps complementary approaches to the problem. The ACMC asks subjects to perform a task they are familiar with and then observes how they solve it. By contrast, the SHAP test assesses the subject's performance on a fixed set of tasks, the score for which is based on the speed of task completion.

More recently, laboratory-based techniques have received growing attention from the research community. These developments, often driven by psychologists and motor control experts, provide a fine-grained insight into the processes underlying prosthesis use. Techniques using motion analysis are now being widely adopted and reveal clear differences in the kinematics of goal-directed behaviours between users of upper limb prostheses and anatomically intact participants. These differences come not only from the limitations of the prosthesis themselves but also from suboptimal training approaches and the tools in this section being used to evaluate both issues. The development of lightweight eye-tracking technologies has led to a number of groups showing how gaze behaviour in prosthesis differs markedly from that seen in anatomically intact participants. Gaze behaviour and analysis of brain activity through EEG studies may offer particular advantages when considering the evaluation of the systems offering sensory feedback.

As the technology of the prosthesis themselves and technologies to track the use of devices in the real world develop, we may see a continuing evolution, or perhaps a revolution in how we evaluate such devices. For instance, if we get to the stage of all prostheses logging details on their use and prosthesis providers and researchers are able to combine these data with other data sets on the properties of the prosthesis itself, the user and their real-world behaviours, we may start to question the value of some of the more basic traditional tests. It may become difficult to justify the time needed to carry out these evaluations, which generally require the clinician/researcher and the participant to be in the same room at the same time. Such evaluations clearly come at a cost, not only the time of the clinician and associated overhead but also, as importantly, the time and cost to the user themselves. In poorer countries, such approaches to evaluation are even more difficult, as the prosthesis users themselves may not be able to afford to travel to the clinic and training for clinicians to carry out some of the tests is expensive and time-consuming (http://acmc.se/how-to-become-an-acmc-rater/). Further, the value of data which relates to a single snapshot in time is open to debate, particularly given the long-term nature of prosthetic rehabilitation.

Nevertheless, real-world approaches are only in their infancy and how researchers, clinicians, users and manufacturers approach the many complex issues which surround the adoption of these techniques will determine whether or not they become a mainstream tool. For instance, issues of privacy and data protection need very careful consideration; legal issues arise over who owns the data which is logged by a prosthetic hand, supplied by a manufacturer, prescribed by a government-run or private clinic and worn by an individual. The interested reader who may want to look into these matters further is referred to recent policy-focused work from the UK [106,107].

Acknowledgements

The writing of this chapter was supported in part by Engineering and Physical Sciences Research Council and National Institute for Health Research, grant number EP/R013985/1.

References

[1]   Lindner HY, Natterlund BS, and Hermansson LM. Upper limb prosthetic outcome measures: review and content comparison based on International Classification of Functioning, Disability and Health. Prosthet Orthot Int. 2010;34(2):109–28.

[2]   Resnik L, Borgia M, Silver B, and Cancio J. Systematic review of measures of impairment and activity limitation for persons with upper limb trauma and amputation. Arch Phys Med Rehabil. 2017;98(9):1863–92 e14.

[3]   World Health Organisation Report. ICF: International Classification of Functioning, Disability and Health; 2001.

[4]   World Health Organisation Report. Towards a common language for Functioning, Disability and Health: ICF Beginner's guide; 2002.

[5]   Hill W, Stavdahl O, Hermansson LM, Kyberd P, Swanson S, and Hubbard S. Functional outcomes in the WHO-ICF model: establishment of the upper limb prosthetic outcome measures group. J Prosthet Orthot. 2009;21(2):5.

[6]   Hill W, Stavdahl O, Hermansson LM, Kyberd P, Swanson S, and Hubbard S. Upper limb prosthetic outcome measures (ULPOM): a working group and their findings. J Prosthet Orthot. 2009;21(2):69–82.

[7]   Hermansson LM, Fisher AG, Bernspang B, and Eliasson AC. Assessment of capacity for myoelectric control: a new Rasch-built measure of prosthetic hand control. J Rehabil Med. 2005;37(3):166–71.

[8]   Hermansson LM, Bodin L, and Eliasson AC. Intra- and inter-rater reliability of the assessment of capacity for myoelectric control. J Rehabil Med. 2006;38(2):118–23.

[9]   Light CM. An intelligent hand prosthesis and evaluation of pathological and prosthetic hand function [Thesis]; 2000.

[10]   Light CM, Chappell PH, and Kyberd PJ. Establishing a standardized clinical assessment tool of pathologic and prosthetic hand function: normative data, reliability, and validity. Arch Phys Med Rehabil. 2002;83(6):776–83.

[11]   Stern EB. Stability of the Jebsen-Taylor Hand Function Test across three test sessions. Am J Occup Ther. 1992;46(7):647–9.

[12]   Vasluian E, Bongers RM, Reinders-Messelink HA, Dijkstra PU, and van der Sluis CK. Preliminary study of the Southampton Hand Assessment Procedure for children and its reliability. BMC Musculoskelet Disord. 2014;15:199.

[13]   Bouwsema H, Kyberd P, Van der Sluis CK, and Bongers RM. Determining skill level in myoelectric prosthesis use with multiple outcome measures. J Rehabil Res Dev. 2012;49.

[14]   Vasluian E, Bongers RM, Reinders-Messelink HA, Burgerhof JG, Dijkstra PU, and van der Sluis CK. Learning effects of repetitive administration of the Southampton Hand Assessment Procedure in novice prosthetic users. J Rehabil Med. 2014;46(8):788–97.

[15]   Burgerhof JG, Vasluian E, Dijkstra PU, Bongers RM, and van der Sluis CK. The Southampton Hand Assessment Procedure revisited: a transparent linear scoring system, applied to data of experienced prosthetic users. J Hand Ther. 2017;30(1):49–57.

[16]   Desrosiers J, Bravo G, Hebert R, Dutil E, and Mercier L. Validation of the Box and Block Test as a measure of dexterity of elderly people: reliability, validity, and norms studies. Arch Phys Med Rehabil. 1994;75(7):751–5.

[17]   Clemente F, D'Alonzo M, Controzzi M, Edin BB, and Cipriani C. Non-invasive, temporally discrete feedback of object contact and release improves grasp control of closed-loop myoelectric transradial prostheses. IEEE Trans Neural Syst Rehabil Eng. 2016;24(12):1314–22.

[18]   Hussaini A and Kyberd P. Refined clothespin relocation test and assessment of motion. Prosthet Orthot Int. 2017;41(3):294–302.

[19]   Kuiken T, Miller L, Lipschutz R, Stubblefield K, and Dumanian G. Prosthetic command signals following targeted hyper-reinnervation nerve transfer surgery. Conf Proc IEEE Eng Med Biol Soc. 2005;7:7652–5.

[20]   Kyberd P, Hussaini A, and Maillet G. Characterisation of the Clothespin Relocation Test as a functional assessment tool. J Rehabil Assist Technol Eng. 2018;5:2055668317750810.

[21]   Hussaini A, Hill W, and Kyberd P. Clinical evaluation of the refined clothespin relocation test: a pilot study. Prosthet Orthot Int. 2019;43(5):485–91.

[22]   Resnik L, Adams L, Borgia M, *et al.* Development and evaluation of the activities measure for upper limb amputees. Arch Phys Med Rehabil. 2013;94(3):488–94 e4.

[23]   Resnik L, Borgia M, and Acluche F. Brief activity performance measure for upper limb amputees: BAM-ULA. Prosthet Orthot Int. 2018;42(1): 75–83.

[24]   Bongers RM, Kyberd P, Bouwsema H, Kenney L, Plettenburg DH, and Van der Sluis CK. Bernstein's levels of construction of movements applied to upper limb prosthetics. J Prosthet Orthot. 2012;24(2):67–76.

[25]   Head J. The effect of socket movement and electrode contact on myoelectric prosthesis control during daily living activities [Thesis]; 2013.

[26]   Chadwell A. The reality of myoelectric prostheses: how do EMG skill, unpredictability of prosthesis response, and delays impact on user functionality and everyday prosthesis use? [Thesis]; 2018.

[27]   Raspopovic S, Capogrosso M, Petrini FM, *et al.* Restoring natural sensory feedback in real-time bidirectional hand prostheses. Sci Transl Med. 2014;6(222):222ra19.

[28]   Valle G, Mazzoni A, Iberite F, *et al.* Biomimetic Intraneural Sensory Feedback Enhances Sensation Naturalness, Tactile sensitivity, and manual dexterity in a bidirectional prosthesis. Neuron. 2018;100(1):37–45 e7.

[29]   Cognolato M, Atzori M, and Muller H. Head-mounted eye gaze tracking devices: an overview of modern devices and recent advances. J Rehabil Assist Technol Eng. 2018;5.

[30]   Sobuh M, Kenney L, Galpin A, Thies S, Kyberd P, and Ruffi R. Coding scheme for characterising gaze behaviour of prosthetic use. In: Myoelectric Control Symposium, New Brunswick, Canada; 2011.

[31]   Land M, Mennie N, and Rusted J. The roles of vision and eye movements in the control of activities of daily living. Perception. 1999;28(11):1311–28.

[32]   Pelz JB and Canosa R. Oculomotor behavior and perceptual strategies in complex tasks. Vision Res. 2001;41(25–26):3587–96.

[33]   Wilson MR, Vine SJ, Bright E, Masters RS, Defriend D, and McGrath JS. Gaze training enhances laparoscopic technical skill acquisition and multi-tasking performance: a randomized, controlled study. Surg Endosc. 2011;25(12):3731–9.

[34]   Bowman MC, Johansson RS, and Flanagan JR. Eye-hand coordination in a sequential target contact task. Exp Brain Res. 2009;195(2):273–83.

[35]   Sailer U, Flanagan JR, and Johansson RS. Eye-hand coordination during learning of a novel visuomotor task. J Neurosci. 2005;25(39):8833–42.

[36]   Sobuh MM, Kenney LP, Galpin AJ, *et al.* Visuomotor behaviours when using a myoelectric prosthesis. J Neuroeng Rehabil. 2014;11:72.

[37]   Chadwell A, Kenney L, Granat MH, *et al.* Upper limb activity in myoelectric prosthesis users is biased towards the intact limb and appears unrelated to goal-directed task performance. Sci Rep. 2018;8(1):11084.

[38]   Chadwell A, Kenney L, Thies S, Galpin A, and Head J. The reality of myoelectric prostheses: understanding what makes these devices difficult for some users to control. Front Neurorobot. 2016;10:7.

[39]   Parr JVV, Vine SJ, Harrison NR, and Wood G. Examining the spatiotemporal disruption to gaze when using a myoelectric prosthetic hand. J Mot Behav. 2018;50(4):416–25.

[40]   Parr JVV, Vine SJ, Wilson MR, Harrison NR, and Wood G. Visual attention, EEG alpha power and T7-Fz connectivity are implicated in prosthetic hand control and can be optimized through gaze training. J Neuroeng Rehabil. 2019;16(1):52.

[41]   Hebert JS, Boser QA, Valevicius AM, *et al.* Quantitative eye gaze and movement differences in visuomotor adaptations to varying task demands among upper-extremity prosthesis users. JAMA Netw Open. 2019;2(9):e1911197.

[42]   Raveh E, Friedman J, and Portnoy S. Evaluation of the effects of adding vibrotactile feedback to myoelectric prosthesis users on performance and visual attention in a dual-task paradigm. Clin Rehabil. 2018;32(10):1308–16.

[43]   Spiers AJ, Resnik L, and Dollar AM. Analyzing at-home prosthesis use in unilateral upper-limb amputees to inform treatment & device design. IEEE Int Conf Rehabil Robot. 2017;2017:1273–80.

[44]   Niechwiej-Szwedo E, Gonzalez D, Nouredanesh M, and Tung J. Evaluation of the leap motion controller during the performance of visually-guided upper limb movements. PLoS One. 2018;13(3):e0193639.

[45]   Bouvier B, Duprey S, Claudon L, Dumas R, and Savescu A. Upper limb kinematics using inertial and magnetic sensors: comparison of sensor-to-segment calibrations. Sensors (Basel). 2015;15(8):18813–33.

[46]   Hodrien A. Exploring factors associated with upper-limb prosthesis embodiment: a mixed-methods approach [Thesis]; 2019.

[47]   Roetenberg D, Slycke PJ, and Veltink PH. Ambulatory position and orientation tracking fusing magnetic and inertial sensing. IEEE Trans Biomed Eng. 2007;54(5):883–90.

[48]   Cappozzo A, Catani F, Croce UD, and Leardini A. Position and orientation in space of bones during movement: anatomical frame definition and determination. Clin Biomech (Bristol, Avon). 1995;10(4): 171–8.

[49]   Wu G, van der Helm FC, Veeger HE, *et al.* ISB recommendation on definitions of joint coordinate systems of various joints for the reporting of human joint motion—Part II: Shoulder, elbow, wrist and hand. J Biomech. 2005;38(5):981–92.

[50]   Resnik L, Acluche F, and Borgia M. The DEKA hand: a multifunction prosthetic terminal device-patterns of grip usage at home. Prosthet Orthot Int. 2018;42(4):446–54.

[51]   Jeannerod M. The timing of natural prehension movements. J Mot Behav. 1984;16(3):235–54.

[52]   Wing AM, Haggard P, and Flanagan JR. Hand and brain. The neurophysiology and psychology of hand movements. Academic Press; 1996.

[53]   Wing AM and Fraser C. The contribution of the thumb to reaching movements. Q J Exp Psychol Sect A – Hum Exp Psychol. 1983;35:297–309.

[54]   Fraser C and Wing AW. A case study of reaching by a user of a manually-operated artificial hand. Prosthet Orthot Int. 1981;5(3):151–6.

[55]   Popat RA, Krebs DE, Mansfield J, *et al.* Quantitative assessment of four men using above-elbow prosthetic control. Arch Phys Med Rehabil. 1993;74(7):720–9.

[56]   Doeringer JA and Hogan N. Performance of above elbow body-powered prostheses in visually guided unconstrained motion tasks. IEEE Trans Biomed Eng. 1995;42(6):621–31.

[57]   Carey SL, Jason Highsmith M, Maitland ME, and Dubey RV. Compensatory movements of transradial prosthesis users during common tasks. Clin Biomech (Bristol, Avon). 2008;23(9):1128–35.

[58]   Carey SL, Dubey RV, Bauer GS, and Highsmith MJ. Kinematic comparison of myoelectric and body powered prostheses while performing common activities. Prosthet Orthot Int. 2009;33(2):179–86.

[59]   Bouwsema H, van der Sluis CK, and Bongers RM. Changes in performance over time while learning to use a myoelectric prosthesis. J Neuroeng Rehabil. 2014;11:16.

[60]   Huinink LH, Bouwsema H, Plettenburg DH, van der Sluis CK, and Bongers RM. Learning to use a body-powered prosthesis: changes in functionality and kinematics. J Neuroeng Rehabil. 2016;13(1):90.

[61] Romkema S, Bongers RM, and van der Sluis CK. Intermanual transfer in training with an upper-limb myoelectric prosthesis simulator: a mechanistic, randomized, pretest-posttest study. Phys Ther. 2013;93(1):22–31.

[62] Romkema S, Bongers RM, and van der Sluis CK. Influence of the type of training task on intermanual transfer effects in upper-limb prosthesis training: A randomized pre-posttest study. PLoS One. 2017;12(11):e0188362.

[63] Murgia A, Kyberd PJ, Chappell PH, and Light CM. Marker placement to describe the wrist movements during activities of daily living in cyclical tasks. Clin Biomech (Bristol, Avon). 2004;19(3):248–54.

[64] Hebert JS and Lewicke J. Case report of modified Box and Blocks test with motion capture to measure prosthetic function. J Rehabil Res Dev. 2012;49(8):1163–74.

[65] Wolpert DM, Diedrichsen J, and Flanagan JR. Principles of sensorimotor learning. Nat Rev Neurosci. 2011;12(12):739–51.

[66] Major MJ, Stine RL, Heckathorne CW, Fatone S, and Gard SA. Comparison of range-of-motion and variability in upper body movements between transradial prosthesis users and able-bodied controls when executing goal-oriented tasks. J Neuroeng Rehabil. 2014;11:132.

[67] Thies SB, Kenney LP, Sobuh M, *et al.* Skill assessment in upper limb myoelectric prosthesis users: validation of a clinically feasible method for characterising upper limb temporal and amplitude variability during the performance of functional tasks. Med Eng Phys. 2017;47:137–43.

[68] Thies SB, Tresadern PA, Kenney LP, *et al.* Movement variability in stroke patients and controls performing two upper limb functional tasks: a new assessment methodology. J Neuroeng Rehabil. 2009;6:2.

[69] Ngan A, Xiao W, Curran PF, *et al.* Functional workspace and patient-reported outcomes improve after reverse and total shoulder arthroplasty. J Shoulder Elbow Surg. 2019;28(11):2121–7.

[70] Chadwell A, Kenney LPJ, Howard D, Ssekitoleko RT, Nakandi BT, and Head J. Evaluating reachable workspace and user control over prehensor aperture for a body-powered prosthesis. IEEE Trans Neural Syst Rehabil Eng (in press).

[71] Fougner A, Scheme E, Chan AD, Englehart K, and Stavdahl O. Resolving the limb position effect in myoelectric pattern recognition. IEEE Trans Neural Syst Rehabil Eng. 2011;19(6):644–51.

[72] Maimon-Mor R. Gesticulation with hand and prosthesis in congenitals one-handers and acquired amputees. In: Trent International Prosthetics Symposium. Salford, UK; 2019.

[73] Choi BCK and Pak AWP. A catalog of biases in questionnaires. Prev Chronic Dis. 2005;2(1):1–13.

[74] Chadwell A, Kenney L, Granat M, Thies S, Head JS, and Galpin A. Visualisation of upper limb activity using spirals: a new approach to the assessment of daily prosthesis usage. Prosthet Orthot Int. 2018;42(1):37–44.

[75] Dobkin BH and Martinez C. Wearable sensors to monitor, enable feedback, and measure outcomes of activity and practice. Curr Neurol Neurosci Rep. 2018;18(12):87.

[76] Dobkin BH. Wearable motion sensors to continuously measure real-world physical activities. Curr Opin Neurol. 2013;26(6):602–8.

[77] Patel S, Park H, Bonato P, Chan L, and Rodgers M. A review of wearable sensors and systems with application in rehabilitation. J Neuroeng Rehabil. 2012;9(1):21.

[78] Rodgers MM, Alon G, Pai VM, and Conroy RS. Wearable technologies for active living and rehabilitation: current research challenges and future opportunities. J Rehabil Assist Technol Eng. 2019;6:2055668319839607.

[79] Vega-Gonzalez A and Granat MH. Continuous monitoring of upper-limb activity in a free-living environment. Arch Phys Med Rehabil. 2005;86(3):541–8.

[80] Chen KY and Bassett JDR. The technology of accelerometry-based activity monitors: current and future. Med Sci Sports Exerc. 2005;37(11 Suppl): S490–500.

[81] Brond JC, Andersen LB, and Arvidsson D. Generating ActiGraph counts from raw acceleration recorded by an alternative monitor. Med Sci Sports Exerc. 2017;49(11):2351–60.

[82] Makin TR, Cramer AO, Scholz J, *et al.* Deprivation-related and use-dependent plasticity go hand in hand. eLife. 2013;2:e01273.

[83] Bailey RR, Klaesner JW, and Lang CE. An accelerometry-based methodology for assessment of real-world bilateral upper extremity activity. PLoS One. 2014;9(7):e103135.

[84] Noorkõiv M, Rodgers H, and Price CI. Accelerometer measurement of upper extremity movement after stroke: a systematic review of clinical studies. J Neuroeng Rehabil. 2014;11(1):144.

[85] Narai E, Hagino H, Komatsu T, and Togo F. Accelerometer-based monitoring of upper limb movement in older adults with acute and subacute stroke. J Geriatr Phys Ther. 2016;39(4):171–7.

[86] Lee SI, Liu X, Rajan S, Ramasarma N, Choe EK, and Bonato P. A novel upper-limb function measure derived from finger-worn sensor data collected in a free-living setting. PLoS One. 2019;14(3):e0212484.

[87] Hayward KS, Eng JJ, Boyd LA, Lakhani B, Bernhardt J, and Lang CE. Exploring the role of accelerometers in the measurement of real world upper-limb use after stroke. Brain Impairment. 2015;17(1):16–33.

[88] Lang CE, Waddell KJ, Klaesner JW, and Bland MD. A method for quantifying upper limb performance in daily life using accelerometers. J. Visualized Exp: JoVE. 2017;(122):55673.

[89] Chadwell A, Kenney L, Granat M, Thies S, Galpin A, and Head J. Upper limb activity of twenty myoelectric prosthesis users and twenty healthy anatomically intact adults. Sci Data. 2019;6(1):199.

[90] Wijndaele K, Westgate K, Stephens SK, *et al.* Utilization and harmonization of adult accelerometry data: review and expert consensus. Med Sci Sports Exerc. 2015;47(10):2129–39.

[91] Knaier R, Höchsmann C, Infanger D, Hinrichs T, and Schmidt-Trucksäss A. Validation of automatic wear-time detection algorithms in a free-living

setting of wrist-worn and hip-worn ActiGraph GT3X+. BMC Public Health. 2019;19(1):244.

[92] Choi L, Liu Z, Matthews CE, and Buchowski MS. Validation of accelerometer wear and nonwear time classification algorithm. Med Sci Sports Exerc. 2011;43(2).

[93] Ahanathapillai V, Amor JD, Tadeusiak M, and James CJ. Wrist-worn accelerometer to detect postural transitions and walking patterns. In: XIII Mediterranean Conference on Medical and Biological Engineering and Computing. Cham: Springer International Publishing. p. 1515–18.

[94] Uswatte G, Foo WL, Olmstead H, Lopez K, Holand A, and Simms LB. Ambulatory monitoring of arm movement using accelerometry: an objective measure of upper-extremity rehabilitation in persons with chronic stroke. Arch Phys Med Rehabil. 2005;86(7):1498–501.

[95] Barreira TV, Zderic TW, Schuna JM, Hamilton MT, and Tudor-Locke C. Free-living activity counts-derived breaks in sedentary time: are they real transitions from sitting to standing? Gait Posture. 2015;42(1):70–2.

[96] Clucas J, White C, Koo B, Milham M, and Klein A. Assessing actimeters for inclusion in the Healthy Brain Network. bioRxiv. 2017:183772.

[97] Chinn N. Wear and use of prostheses in sport by adolescents with upper limb absence: a mixed methods study [Thesis]; 2019.

[98] Chadwell A, Diment L, Micó-Amigo M, *et al.* Technology for monitoring everyday prosthesis use: a systematic review. J Neuroeng Rehabil. 2020;17(1):93.

[99] Biddiss EA and Chau TT. Upper limb prosthesis use and abandonment: a survey of the last 25 years. Prosthet Orthot Int. 2007;31(3):236–57.

[100] Major MJ and Fey NP. Considering passive mechanical properties and patient user motor performance in lower limb prosthesis design optimization to enhance rehabilitation outcomes. Phys Ther Rev. 2017;22(3–4):1–15.

[101] Atzori M, Gijsberts A, Castellini C, *et al.* Electromyography data for non-invasive naturally-controlled robotic hand prostheses. Sci Data. 2014;1:140053.

[102] Ottenbacher KJ, Graham JE, and Fisher SR. Data science in physical medicine and rehabilitation: opportunities and challenges. Phys Med Rehabil Clin N Am. 2019;30(2):459–71.

[103] NIH. NIH strategic plan for data science; 2018. Available from: https://datascience.nih.gov/strategicplan.

[104] Hicks JL, Althoff T, Sosic R, *et al.* Best practices for analyzing large-scale health data from wearables and smartphone apps. NPJ Digit Med. 2019;2:45.

[105] Smit G and Plettenburg DH. Efficiency of voluntary closing hand and hook prostheses. Prosthet Orthot Int. 2010;34(4):411–27. Available from: https://www.ncbi.nlm.nih.gov/pubmed/20849359.

[106] Royal Academy of Medical Sciences Report. Human enhancement and the future of work; 2012.

[107] Royal Society Report. iHuman perspective: neural interfaces; 2019.

Chapter 4
Magnetomyography
*Siming Zuo[1], Kianoush Nazarpour[2], Martina Gerken[3]
and Hadi Heidari[1]*

Signals produced by skeletal muscle can be utilised for monitoring and treatment of different movement and neurological disorders. The study of muscle function through measurement of biomagnetic signals is called magnetomyography (MMG). However, the level of biomagnetic signals is extremely small and developing highly sensitive sensors to detect them is outstandingly challenging. Current technologies for detection of such weak biomagnetic signals are bulky, costly and hospital-based. The research findings are yet to develop miniaturised, sensitive and low-cost MMG sensors. This chapter describes the state-of-the-art magnetic sensing technologies that have the potential to realise a low profile and possibly implantable MMG sensor.

The MMG method is the measurement and study of the magnetic manifestation of muscle activity, first formally proposed in 1972 [1]. They defined the magneto-myogram signal to be a recording of one component of the magnetic field vector versus time, where the magnetic field at the point of measurement is due to currents generated by skeletal muscle. Over the past four decades, the fidelity, temporal and spatial resolution of macroscopic and non-invasive detection of biomagnetic signals have progressed significantly. Examples include the magnetocardiography (MCG) and magnetoencephalography (MEG) methods, evidenced by a significant difference in the number of publications since the 1970s, as shown in Figure 4.1(a), when compared to MMG studies. It clearly shows that research in the electromyography (EMG) field far exceeds the MMG. We discuss the advantages and challenges of MMG for measuring magnetic fields from skeletal muscles. Emerging sensor technologies are presented that might provide valuable and feasible data for a better understanding of skeletal muscle physiology in the near future.

The correspondence between the MMG method and its electrical counterpart, that is, the EMG technique [2], stems directly from the Maxwell–Ampère law, as shown in Figure 4.1(b). However, the ease at which the EMG signal can be recorded and the similarity between the temporal and spectral characteristics of the MMG and EMG signals have encouraged the academic and clinical communities to utilise the

[1]James Watt School of Engineering, University of Glasgow, Glasgow, UK
[2]The University of Edinburgh, Edinburgh, UK
[3]Institute of Electrical and Information Engineering, Kiel University, Kiel, Germany

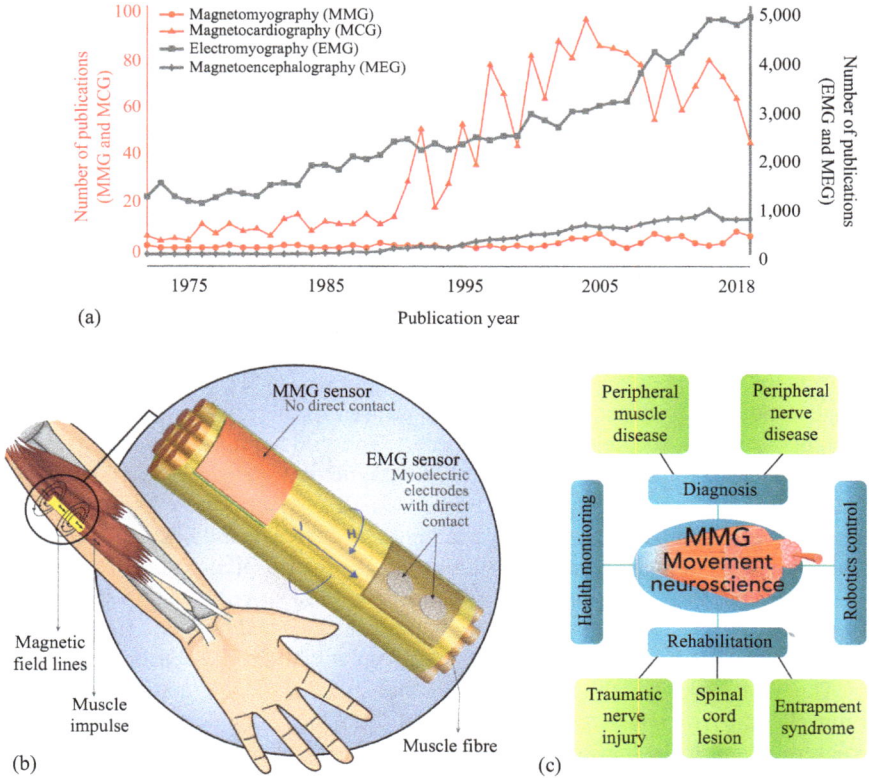

Figure 4.1   (a) Number of published papers that used MMG, MCG, EMG and
MEG methods since 1970. Data was extracted from Web of Science
by searching keywords: magnetomyography, magnetomyogram,
magnetocardiography, electromyography and
magnetoencephalography; (b) schematic of the magnetic versus
electric approaches to sensing muscle activity; (c) potential
application of MMG for diagnosis and rehabilitation of
movement disorder, health monitoring and robotics control

EMG method preferentially. As such the progress of the MMG method has been rather slow. Biomagnetic signals are typically weak, a million times weaker than the geomagnetic field. They can be polluted by environmental magnetic noise readily. Hence, most biomagnetic sensing studies take place in magnetically shielded rooms.

Two key drivers for the development of the MMG method are as follows [3]: (1) poor spatial resolution of the EMG signals when recorded non-invasively on the skin and (2) poor biocompatibility of the implantable EMG sensors due to the metal–tissue interface. Implanted MMG sensors have the potential to address both shortcomings concurrently because (1) the size of the magnetic field increased significantly with the reduced distance between the origin and the sensor, thereby with MMG spatial resolution is uplifted; (2) the MMG sensors do not need electrical contacts to record, hence if fully packaged with biocompatible materials or polymers, they can improve long-term biocompatibility.

Nowadays, the MMG signals have become an important indicator for medical diagnosis, rehabilitation, health monitoring and robotics control (Figure 4.1(c)) [3]. Such magnetic information about physiological phenomena is directly associated with human health and well-being. Recent advances in wearable technology have paved a way to remotely and continuously record and diagnose individuals' disease on the peripheral muscle and the peripheral nerve [13].

It is important for each individual to understand their physiological and health status by analysing biosignals. Then, appropriate treatments can be provided in a timely manner. Motivated by exploring the electrophysiological behaviour of the uterus prior to childbirth, previous MMG in use is mainly focused on health monitoring during pregnancy [14]. The produced spatial–temporal map of the muscles will provide a better understanding of the process of labour. In addition, the MMG has the potential to be used in rehabilitation such as the traumatic nerve injury, spinal cord lesion and entrapment syndrome [15]. One of the most important research areas in the MMG is to develop rehabilitation robotics where human–machine interfaces assist the disabled with limb difference to perform essential activities of daily living. Currently, the widely and practically used hand prosthesis feed-forward control is only driven by EMG signals, sensing changes of electric potentials from the skin surface of an amputee's stump due to the muscle contractions and allowing the user to operate the prosthesis. However, for the problem of feed-forward control of hand prostheses, whether via pattern recognition [16,17] or abstract control [18–20], the EMG is far from achieving an optimal solution due to the lack of spatial resolution [21]. The MMG becomes an efficient and robust alternative [3,22] for upper limb prosthesis control, enabling algorithms to extract features from the MMG signals that can efficiently and compactly represent information relevant to muscle movement.

The integrated magnetic sensing technology has attracted interest as evidenced by a growing number of applications. For their adoption, it is critical to enhance the micro-dimensional detection sensitivity and the functional robustness of the sensors as required in real-time sensing and processing applications. The development of miniaturised biomagnetic sensing methods would constitute an important step towards the wider appreciation of biomagnetism. Figure 4.2 illustrates the progress pathway of the biomagnetic sensors from superconducting quantum interference devices (SQUIDs) [1], atom magnetometer [4], neuromagnetic current probe [5], optically pumped magnetometers (OPMs) [7] to spintronic devices [8] with the state-of-the-art examples and integrated microneedles [10–12].

The era of spin-based sensors began with the invention of the giant magnetoresistive (GMR) effect which concerns the intrinsic spin of the electron and its associated magnetic moment, in addition to its fundamental electronic charge. The magnetoresistive (MR) effect is observed in artificial thin-film materials composed of alternate ferromagnetic (FM) and nonmagnetic layers. In principle, spintronic sensors can accommodate compact sensors with sizes comparable to or smaller than that of the

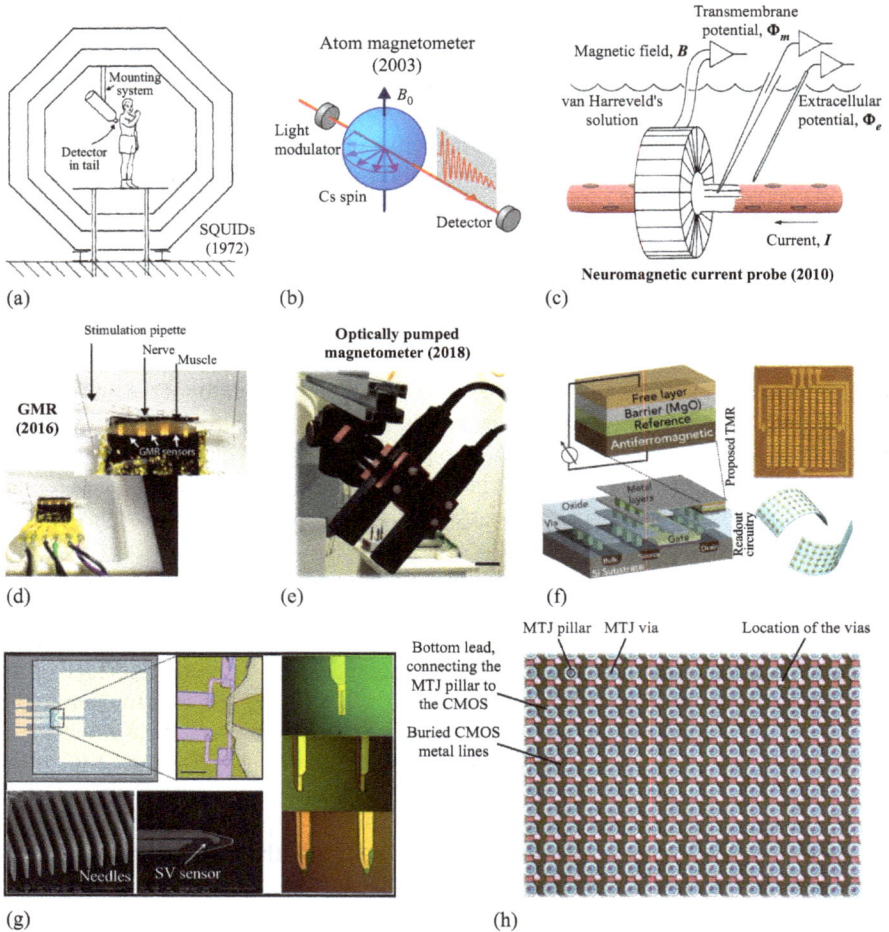

Figure 4.2   Overview of weak biomagnetic detection in skeletal muscle using MMG, showing the miniaturisation pathway from bulky SQUIDs to spintronic nanoscale devices: (a) SQUIDs [1]; (b) atom magnetometer [4]; (c) neuromagnetic current probe [5]; (d) GMR [6]; (e) optical pumped magnetometer [7]; (f) spintronic sensors [8] with flexible TMR [9]; state-of-the-art: (g) MR microneedles [10–12]; (h) TMR array integrated with the standard CMOS technology [8]

conventional SQUIDs for MMG. Yet, there are significant performance trade-offs in exploiting these technologies, particularly in terms of signal-to-noise ratio (SNR). Over the last decade, significant work has been performed to improve the detection range of spintronics-based sensors to sub-pico-tesla (pT)/Hz$^{1/2}$ levels [8], for instance by utilising the tunnelling magnetoresistive (TMR) sensors. We intend to provide a perspective of miniature magnetic sensors for biomagnetic signal detection and demonstrate the feasibility of integrated TMR sensors for MMG applications. First, the magnetic field generated by a typical skeletal muscle is modelled to provide a context in terms of the size of the MMG signals. Then, we review the state of the art in sub-pT magnetic sensing technologies to provide guidance for the future development of an integrated MMG technology. In addition, we present simulation data supporting the view that integrated complementary metal-oxide-semiconductor (CMOS) compatible spintronic sensors and other candidates can be utilised for MMG sensing. We then discuss several technical challenges related to biomagnetic sensing such as nulling the Earth's magnetic field and movement artefacts. Finally, we posit that with addressing these technical challenges, the development of novel MMG sensing methods can facilitate a scientific revolution by providing additional details about the mechanics of the skeletal muscles and also feature a breakthrough in human–machine interfacing applications.

4.1 MMG signal modelling

The magnitude of the MMG signal depends on several parameters. For instance, the distance between the source of the signal and the sensor can change the magnitude from nano-tesla, when the MMG signals are recorded for isolated muscle fibres or with an implanted sensor below the skin, to pT, when sensors are placed on the skin, outside of the body [15]. In the following, we provide a simple model to investigate the effect of the distance between the sensor and a single fibre on the magnitude of the MMG signals, depending on bundle and radial and axial conductivities of a muscle bundle. Figure 4.3(a) illustrates this model.

The magnetic field produced by an action potential travelling in a single muscle fibre, Figure 4.3(a), can be calculated using the approach developed by Roth and Wikswo [23]. Their method presents the advantage of using Ampère's law, which allows disentangling the contributions to the magnetic field due to the currents present in each region of the system, including the fibres, the bundle, the sheath of connective tissue and the bath. We generalised this model to the case of a muscle composed of several fibres. The geometry of the muscle is depicted in Figure 4.3(b) and a set of parameters describing the muscle bundle following the settings used in [24].

The muscle fibre was modelled as a cylindrical cable composed of 1,200 compartments of 10 μm length and 50 μm diameter. A cylindrical fibre of diameter $a = 50$ μm was placed at distance t from the centre of the bundle. The bundle had a diameter $b = 150$ and 50 μm diameter fibres separated by a 10 μm interstitial space and was surrounded by a sheath with thickness $\delta = 10$ μm. All simulations were performed with NEURON [25] and MATLAB® (MathWorks 2017a). The full expressions of calculation and boundary conditions are detailed by Roth and Wikswo [23] and were solved using standard Python routines for a system of linear scalar equations. Here, the parameters were adjusted to characterise the different currents in order to reproduce the action potential shape recorded on the soleus skeletal muscle cells under

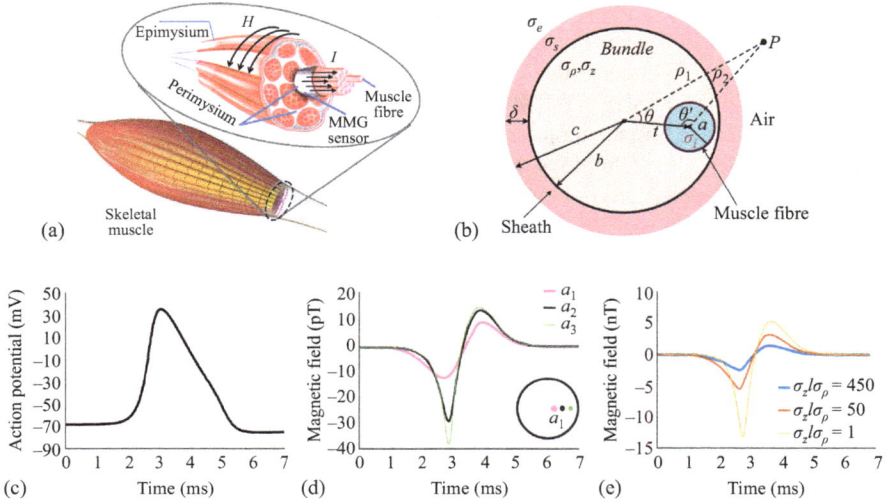

Figure 4.3   (a) *Microstructure of muscle (image is taken from https://www.vcg.com/); (b) scheme of the muscle model; (c) an action potential of the skeletal muscle fibre; (d) net magnetic field of a single fibre depending on its position inside the bundle. This net field contains different magnetic field components due to the currents flowing in the fibre (B_i), the bundle (B_b), the sheath (B_s) and the saline (B_e). (e) Magnetic field generated by the entire muscle at 30 μm from the surface for different values of the ratio σ_z/σ_ρ ($\sigma_z = 5/\Omega/m$), where the axial and radial conductivities are σ_z and σ_ρ*

floating electrode recording conditions. Using this model and the transmembrane potential, as shown in Figure 4.3(c), the x, y and z components of the magnetic action field at an observation point P, outside the muscle bundle, were calculated. As shown in Figure 4.3(d), the net magnetic field was calculated for a single fibre located at distances d from the centre of the bundle. We studied the behaviour of the magnetic field due to the different currents as a function of axial and radial conductivities of the muscle bundle, that is, σ_z and σ_ρ, respectively. As the ratio σ_z/σ_ρ increases, the shielding effect is more prominent, and hence the magnitude of the magnetic signal is decreased. In other words, when a fibre is close to the centre of the bundle, the current in the bundle shields the generated magnetic field. Finally, Figure 4.3(e) shows the total magnetic field B_{total} modelled at point P and the relative contributions due to the intracellular current B_i, the currents flowing in the bundle B_b, in the sheath B_s and in the external saline B_e. It should be noted that contributions from saline and sheath currents are much smaller than that of bundle currents. As such, extracellular bundle currents can be considered as the primary source of shielding [23].

4.2 MMG sensing technologies

Magnetic sensors convert the magnetic field into corresponding measurable electrical signals such as voltage and current. The frequency and magnitude of magnetic signals generated by the human body are demonstrated in Figure 4.4 [26]. In general, there are two categories of biomagnetic sensors: (1) sensitive only to the strength of the magnetic field, including devices such as OPM and atomic magnetometer that measure the magnitude of the magnetic field in the femto-tesla range [4,7]; (2) sensitive to the strength and direction of the magnetic field, including SQUIDs, Hall sensors, MR, magneto-electric (ME) and magneto-impedance sensors, conventional superconducting coils and fluxgates. These vectorial sensors integrate multiple single-component sensors which are placed on linearly independent directions. Some integrated vector magnetometer designs use micromachined electromechanical systems technology to obtain linear independence and some designs use in-plane Hall sensors and instrumentation amplifiers to obtain all components of the magnetic field.

A special categorisation of magnetic sensors considers whether the magnetic field causes electrons to move through various layers of semiconductor material within the sensor, the so-called magneto-transport effect. Examples of technologies that benefit from the magneto-transport phenomenon include Hall probes and MR, ME and magneto-impedance sensors. In the following, we first briefly review the main features of the conventional SQUIDs, fluxgate sensors and the recently developed OPMs. We then compare them with the magneto-transport devices. Table 4.1 summarises this comparison [3].

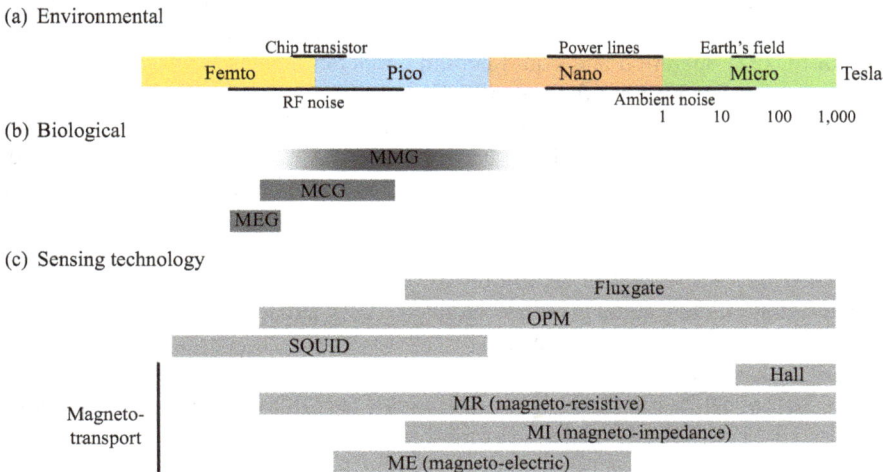

Figure 4.4   A summary of the strength of various example magnetic signals in comparison to biological signals and LODs of existing magnetic sensing technologies

*Table 4.1   Main magnetic sensing technologies and their properties. $\sqrt{}$: Ideal,
●: Acceptable, ▲: Marginally Acceptable, ×: Difficult*

	Sensitivity	Spatial res.	Freq.	Miniaturisation	Portability	Cost
OPM	●	●	DC	×	×	▲
GMI	▲	●	DC-10 kHz	$\sqrt{}$	$\sqrt{}$	$\sqrt{}$
ME	●	●	DC-MHz	●	$\sqrt{}$	$\sqrt{}$
Coil	●	$\sqrt{}$	AC	×	●	$\sqrt{}$
Fluxgate	●	$\sqrt{}$	DC-5 kHz	$\sqrt{}$	$\sqrt{}$	●
SQUID	$\sqrt{}$	●	DC-100 kHz	×	×	×
MR	●	$\sqrt{}$	DC-GHz	$\sqrt{}$	$\sqrt{}$	$\sqrt{}$

Although the MMG signal is ultra-low in the scale of pico (10^{-12}) to femto (10^{-15}) tesla [15], decreasing strongly with the distance between the sensor and the muscle fibre, non-invasive MMG measurements with magnetometers can offer vector information, long-term biocompatibility with tissue, a higher SNR and better positioning and fast screening of sensors without electrical contacts, where the magnetic sensors can be fully packaged within a fully biocompatible material. However, the high cost and cumbersome traditional MMG devices, SQUIDs, block the spread of such magnetic diagnostic techniques. The SQUID is the most sensitive device so far with femto-tesla sensing accuracy and the possibility to achieve atto-tesla (10^{-18} T) detection with averaging, widely used in many biomedical applications for sensing MCG and MEG signals. Nevertheless, such sensitivity levels of SQUIDs require them to remain in a magnetically shielded room that is equipped with an appropriate cooling system for [27] operation at a liquid-helium temperature of 4.2 K [22]. In addition, these requirements increase the cost of SQUID sensors significantly.

Recording of the MMG signal is a challenging task [15] because its magnitude can be as low as hundreds of fT/Hz$^{1/2}$ between 10 and 100 Hz. The main challenges of MMG measurements stem from the dimension, detection limit and SNR of magnetic sensors, since the amplitude of the Earth's magnetic field is about five million times larger, and environmental noise from power lines can reach a nano-tesla level. Over the past decade, a variety of small-dimension and room-temperature sensors have been developed. They enjoy great potential to achieve sufficient sensitivity and to be implemented very close to human skin.

OPMs have improved significantly in limit of detection (LOD) in recent years. LOD values of below 100 fT/Hz$^{1/2}$ have been achieved [28]. They have been employed to measure MMG signals of the hand muscles, evoked by electrical stimulation of the nerves. The OPM sensors, as shown in Figure 4.5(a), can evaluate the transmission of laser light to detect the local magnetic field. Handheld and easy-to-use OPM sensors have recently become commercially available by competing manufacturers, e.g. QuSpin Inc., FieldLine Inc. and Twinleaf. Development of such sensors with small profile enables fitment in wearable devices such as a helmet [28]. Benefiting

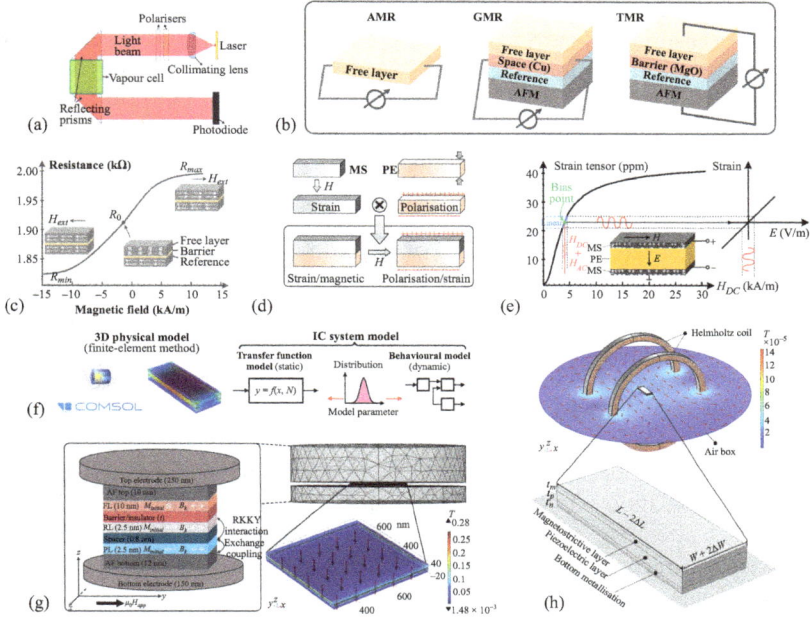

Figure 4.5   Thin-film biomagnetic sensors: (a, b) the typical structures of OPM
[23] and MR sensors; (c) TMR sensor transfer curve and
magnetisation orientations; (d) the principle of ME sensor; (e) the
dynamic small-signal regime; (f) the 3D physical and IC system
models; (g) an MTJ stack layout used for FEM simulations and
orientation of simulation input vectors relative to coordinate axes;
(h) the simulation result of uniform magnetic field distribution in the
central x–y plane under the excitation of a pair of Helmholtz coils

from the quantum sensing technology, these devices approach the same sensitivity
level that cryocooled SQUID offer, but in room temperature. Unfortunately, current
experiments based on OPMs for MMG sensing are conducted in heavily shielded
rooms, which are expensive and bulky for personal daily use. In addition, it is still
rather complex in the sensor setup and the operation. Fluxgate sensors and giant mag-
netoimpedance (GMIs) sensors are well-established sensor concepts and both have
similar dimensions, frequency ranges and LODs at low pT/Hz$^{1/2}$ ranges [29,30].
Although they have small size and can be placed closer to the object, the worse LOD
compared to OPMs and SQUIDs makes them not ideal candidates for the MMG measurement. In addition, the fluxgates have a limited dynamic range and manufacturing
is complex. Thus, they are very expensive to use.

With the emergence of the technologies that utilise the magneto-transport phenomenon, the field of magnetic sensing has been revolutionised [8]. Sensors with

multilayered structure offer a small footprint and the possibility of integration into CMOS. The sensitivity of current magneto-transport sensors is still lower than bulky SQUIDs and rival the performance that OPMs offer. But unlike SQUIDs and flux-gates, they do not require any special operating conditions in terms of temperature. As such they are rather inexpensive and low power.

4.2.1   Magnetoresistive (MR) sensors

Magnetic sensors based on the MR effect have been widely explored over the past years for detection of pT magnetic fields at room temperature. Supplied with a direct current (DC), they convert an external magnetic field directly to a resistance. These sensors use FM and nonmagnetic materials whose magnetisation aligns with the external field to maximise their resistance dynamic range, including anisotropic magnetoresistance (AMR), GMR and TMR. Figure 4.5(b) shows their general structures.

The MR sensors can measure ultra-low magnetic fields at room temperature, while the cost of a typical sensor is approximately a tenth of the cost of a SQUID. They not only offer a wide dynamic range to be hardly affected by disturbance magnetic fields – hence operating with basic shielding – but also have excellent temperature characteristics, which means resistance variations due to the temperature change are negligible through Wheatstone bridge configuration. In addition, the full compatibility between the novel spintronic sensors based on the MR effect and the conventional silicon technology opens a realm of opportunities in which MR sensors can be fabricated with high yields in sub-millimetre diameter substrates. In other words, these sensors can be fully integrated with standard CMOS chips with the readout circuitry to ultimately achieve on-chip signal processing, amplification and noise cancellation.

During the early stage, applications of GMR sensors focused on industry field [31], especially for information storage. Over the past several decades, however, extensive research activities have been triggered to exploit the potentials of integrated GMR sensors in weak biomagnetic detection [32,33]. GMR sensors can realise reliable size-independent magnetic signal detection in the sub-nano-tesla range at room temperature using micron-sized structures. Without increasing the cost or complicating structures, they bring aggregative performance improvements in the fabrication process, structure size, anti-noise ability and sensitivity, benefiting from multiple technologies and the inherent properties of the GMR effect. Recently, they have been implemented in the MEG [34] and MCG [35] measurements, in which the sensitivity of the GMR sensors is now approaching that of SQUIDs and paves the way for spintronic devices for functional sensing and imaging of the body activities. Smart GMR system can also be integrated with multiple components of silicon-based circuits on small platforms such as lab-on-a-chip devices, signal processing and communication modules. It will simplify the on-chip amplification and noise cancellation difficulty and reduce power consumption to sub-mW. Such miniaturised structures without sensitivity loss improve spatial resolution in weak biomagnetic field sensing due to real-time and multimode process based on high compatibility with standard CMOS processes [36]. A successful study shows biocompatible sensors based on GMR spintronics to simultaneously and locally record the magnetic fields from action potentials in a mouse muscle in vitro [34]. The GMR-based micro-probes permitted the miniaturisation and shaping required for in vivo/vitro magnetophysiology and represented a new fundamental tool to investigate the local sources of neuronal magnetic activity [37].

Recent developments in physics and materials promise a new class of solid-state spintronic sensors based on the TMR effect, which occurs in magnetic tunnel junctions (MTJs). These sensors can be faster, more reliable and of lower power than the existing spintronic sensors. The impact of the TMR sensors on the field of spintronics has hugely advanced [8], mainly due to the large magnitude of the observed magnetoresistances at room temperature that surpasses that of the AMR and GMR sensors. The TMR effect has been known since 1975 [38] and is observed on FM spin tunnelling junctions consisting of FM-insulator-FM layers. Figure 4.5(c) shows the basic structure of a TMR-based sensor and its transfer curve, which represents the output resistance dependence on the magnetic field signal directly. The magnetic orientation of the pinned layer is fixed, while the magnetic orientation of the free layer will change in accordance with the direction of the external magnetic field. The electrical resistance of the TMR sensor changes along with this change in the free layer. When the magnetisations are at a perpendicular angle, the resistance is at a value halfway between R_H and R_L. This is often an ideal angle and field for the 'operating point' of a sensor because the linear behaviour occurs at this point. Classical physics predicts that there should be no current flowing through the insulating barrier when a voltage is applied to the FM electrodes on both sides of an MTJ. However, when the insulating barrier is ultra-thin, in the scale of a few nanometres, a quantum tunnelling effect may take place in the junction, which allows electrons to transfer from one FM layer to the other. With a bias voltage, the MTJ exhibits electrical conducting properties, and its electrical resistance varies as a function of the magnetic field strength over a certain field range.

The TMR sensors are gradually replacing the GMR devices because of their higher MR ratio and better SNR. In addition, TMR sensors have a tuneable response and adjustable operation range. Therefore, they are ideal candidates for applications in which pT-level operation at room temperature, small footprint and cost are key factors. Multiple TMR sensors are compatible with standard silicon-integrated circuit technology [8], allowing for large-scale fabrication and closed-packed implementations, which is ideal for portable solutions.

4.2.2 Magnetoelectric sensors

Thin-film magnetoelectric (ME) sensors have increasingly drawn attention over the past decade due to their small dimensions and the possibility of integration with microelectromechanical systems. The engineered ME composites now are promising candidates as magnetic field sensors in unshielded environments and at room temperature [39]. The ME sensors offer passive detection, high sensitivity, large effect enhancement at mechanical resonances and large linear dynamic range. In the past decades, this type of sensors has achieved a high $pT/Hz^{1/2}$ LOD range at low frequencies [40]. In addition, the LODs at a mechanical resonance state are already below fluxgate sensors and GMIs. To measure low-frequency magnetic signals, magnetic frequency conversion techniques with modulation coils should be implemented, to enable to measure at virtually any frequency outside the mechanical resonance. The noise performance over a frequency range of 100 Hz can be interpreted as the LOD as a function of frequency. The resonance curve of the sensor is compensated by digital equalisation. For example, recently, the ME sensors have been used for MCG measurements with a volunteer inside a magnetically shielded room to remove the large unwanted magnetic background noise [41]. Although the sensitivity is not as high as that of the SQUID, the ME sensors show significant superiority in simple preparation and low cost. Furthermore, the ME sensors are CMOS compatible and have a higher detection sensitivity, compared to other integrated semiconductor magnetic sensors such as Hall sensors. We previously developed a high-performance Hall sensor integrated with its readout circuit in CMOS technology [22]. However, it requires a highly stable DC power supply to excite the Hall effect and a complex interface circuit to process collected weak Hall voltages under surrounding noise. The spintronic sensors, especially our previous design of the TMR sensor [42], offer high sensitivity for biosensing applications. Still, both a single TMR sensor and a sensor array (typical configuration is a Wheatstone bridge) are active, requiring stable power supply and suffering higher $1/f$ noise. One of the advantages of the ME sensor is that it is driven with a magnetic bias and will generate the output voltage by itself, indicating it is a passive two-terminal element, which can minimise the size of an ME measurement system without external batteries and achieve a low power consumption. Therefore, the ME sensor could also be a suitable alternative for the MMG measurement with the relatively low operating costs. Moreover, an array of the ME sensors can be built up and placed closer to the measured muscle due to their very small dimension.

The ME effect is a phenomenon in which an electric polarisation is generated by a magnetic field. As illustrated in Figure 4.5(d), in composite ME materials it is a result of the product of the magnetostrictive (MS) effect in the magnetic phase and the piezoelectric (PE) effect in the piezoelectric phase. Then, the ME voltage coefficient, α_{ME}, can be expressed as [39]

$$\alpha_{ME} = \frac{\text{mechanical}}{\text{magnetic}} \times \frac{\text{electric}}{\text{mechanical}} = \frac{\partial \epsilon}{\partial H} \times \frac{\partial \sigma}{\partial \epsilon} \times \frac{\partial P}{\partial \sigma} \tag{4.1}$$

which depends upon the materials combination, interface quality, DC magnetic bias and operational mode [40].

The dynamic small-signal principle of the ME sensor is demonstrated in Figure 4.5(e). Applying a magnetic field, H, along the length direction of the ME composite, the MS layer will elongate along the field direction and generate a strain tensor ϵ because of magnetostriction, which will transfer a stress tensor σ to the PE layer, where the polarisation, P, is changed with stress. Therefore, there is a potential difference induced in the PE layer due to the transverse response. To enhance the response or increase sensor sensitivity, a low harmonic magnetic field is commonly employed using an exciting coil surrounding the sensor operated at a mechanical resonance frequency. Thus, the thin-film ME sensors can transform magnetic fields into a measurable polarisation via a mechanical coupling of the MS and PE layers. Such strong ME coupling provides greater flexibility for applications as biosensing devices. Since the one-end of the sensor is fixed, for cantilever ME sensors with length $\gg$ width $\gg$ height, it only has one sensitivity direction to avoid a cross-sensitivity problem. It is noted that assembled sensor arrays are a common method utilised for the vector measurements. The state-of-the-art magnetic field sensors based on thin-film ME composites have demonstrated their potential of sub-pT/Hz$^{1/2}$ magnetic noise level at room temperature under certain conditions [40].

4.2.3 Device modelling and implementation

Testing all combinations of structures and materials for new sensors in the fabrication is expensive and time-consuming. Therefore, accurate and reliable simulation techniques are employed to evaluate the behaviours of certain material combinations and sensor geometries.

4.2.3.1 Tunnelling magnetoresistive sensors

The optimisation of materials and the fabrication process to obtain high MR ratio is still a challenging task. Modelling of MTJ devices based on MgO barrier shows higher MR ratio in comparison to the Al_2O_3 barrier devices [42] where we showed that such simulation results and parameters can be extracted and imported to the Cadence Spectre simulator for integration with a CMOS-based readout circuit. Therefore, we believe that the TMR sensors with the MgO barrier are highlighted as the most competitive sensors that could achieve sub-pT detection at room temperature and low-frequency domain. Traditionally, 3D physical models are studied separately in finite-element method (FEM) software, and then simulation results will be sent to a signal flow IC system model with a fixed configuration. This approach will bring about that any change in the configuration requires an extra round of FEM simulations. Therefore, a barrier is formed between the physical model and the integrated circuit system model (see Figure 4.5(f)). To avoid this situation, an MR sensor compact model is developed. Here, an FEM model of the magnetic sensor is created and simulated in COMSOL Multiphysics®. The parameters of the FEM model were then exported into Cadence using Verilog-A language, which connects both models for integrated chip designers so that the model can be designed and integrated into a standard CMOS readout circuit. This setting offered the possibility of including circuits for on-chip amplification, signal processing and noise cancellation.

Our recent work proposed FEM simulations of magnetic biosensors and evaluation of their performance in terms of the TMR ratio and linearisation range [43]. The MTJ stack is shown in Figure 4.5(g), which is a current-perpendicular-to-plane multilayer between two leads in with double-exchange electrodes, consisting of bottom antiferromagnet (AFM), pinned layer, spacer, reference layer, barrier, sensing layer and top-AFM. The 3D structure of the MTJ can be divided into small elements with tetrahedral meshes of user-defined sizes. This FEM model is used to estimate the current distribution of the MTJ with different strength of the magnetic field. In addition, the computational meshes with different resolutions can reduce discretisation errors and an enlarged view of the thin-film structure where the colour legend shows magnetic flux density and the arrow represents the direction of the current density. Compared with achievable TMR responses with fabricated sensors [11,44], our recent modelling results show a higher TMR ratio and better linearisation [42].

To minimise undesired effects, especially for temperature drifts in sensing, a Wheatstone bridge (Figure 4.6(a)) configuration with four TMR elements can be utilised [45]. The integrations of the MR sensors are demonstrated with state-of-the-art examples [8,11,12]. The full compatibility between the TMR technologies and the silicon industry opens a new way of the system miniaturisation. One of the important biosensing applications is achieved by the integration of an array of MR sensors on sharp, machined probes. They enjoy the ability to measure directly and locally the magnetic fields related to human activity such as brain and heart at room temperature. The recent in vitro measurement is for brain activity monitoring upon electrical stimulation. It requires special sensor geometries where sharp probes incorporated single or large arrays of TMR sensors with microelectrodes microfabricated in the same fabrication process. Integrating state-of-the-art MgO-based TMR sensors into Si needles, it can be used as a miniature tool for the biomagnetic sensing at very weak fields level, especially pico-to-femto-tesla with a low-frequency domain. Currently, multidimension technology has achieved the sensitivity of 100–300 mV/V/Oe in a larger prototype commercial TMR sensors, TMR9001/9002. With continuous research, pT-level detection has been achieved at room temperature.

Moreover, recent progress achieved the integration of functional MR sensors with flexible materials for new devices and applications [9]. The MR technology has pushed the integration limits towards stretchable substrates to form a flexible and bendable sensor solution. Motivated by the continued researches for wearable and implantable sensing, microfabricated devices on flexible substrates can bend and conform to the non-planar geometries. The TMR sensors were measured onto ultrathin flexible silicon membrane where the TMR sensor maintains its MR ratio when compared with rigid substrates such as Si or glass. This flexible MgO-barrier device enjoys flexibility, thermal stability, chemical resistance, high mechanical modulus and biocompatibility. Figure 4.6(b) shows an example of monolithic integration on standard CMOS with fabricated TMR sensor with its readout circuitry from the Iberian Nanotechnology Laboratory [8].

A real-time miniaturised readout system for newly developed TMR sensors is illustrated in Figure 4.6(c), which comprises a Wheatstone bridge configuration with four TMR sensors, as well as its analogue front-end (AFE) and digital back-end signal processing units which are needed for generating selected useful information from the measured MMG signals. First of all, the Wheatstone bridge can operate in the voltage-mode or the current-mode by using two toggle switches as selectors. The stable power supplies are provided by a voltage regulator and a current generator. The proposed AFE includes a transimpedance amplifier (TIA), an instrumentation amplifier, bandpass filters, a programmable gain amplifier, an analogue multiplexer, micro control unit, which includes an analogue-to-digital converter. Finally, the signals are transmitted

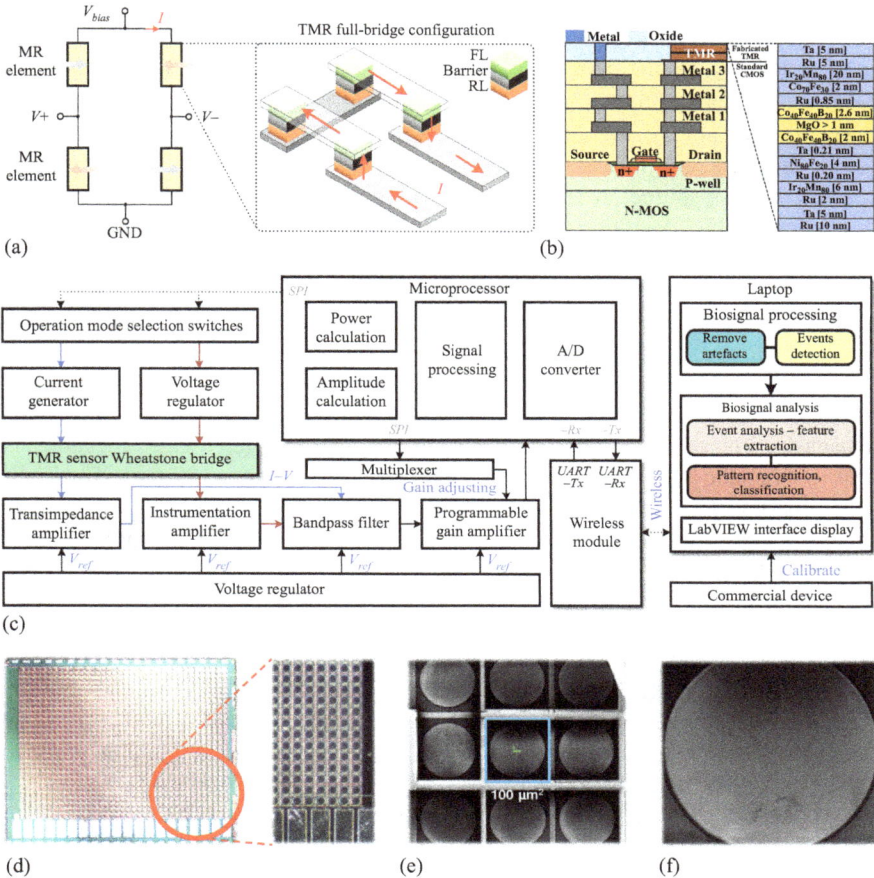

Figure 4.6 (a) Schematic diagram of the biomagnetic field measurement system using TMR sensors where four integrated TMR sensors are connected in a bridge; (b) monolithic integration of the TMR sensor on standard CMOS with its readout circuitry; (c) a block diagram of a general processing chain for TMR sensors that can be utilised for MMG applications; (d) microscope and zoom-in pictures of the TMR sensor array in post-cleaning; (e) a zoom-in picture with a size of 100 μm² per TMR element; (f) a single TMR element

through a wireless module and then extracted, classified and displayed in a LabVIEW interface on the laptop. Our previously ultra-low noise current source and TIA are utilised to bias and amplify from bridge signals with external noise filtering switched capacitors [45], allowing CMOS integration of TMR sensors without decreasing the measurement resolution.

In particular, the advantages of scaling and higher density integration must be balanced against the requirements of low noise design, uniform power density, surface temperature distribution, better component matching and immunity to parameter variations [46]. In addition, the spatial resolution can be improved by scaling an array of sensors that can measure the biomagnetic field from different points. To enhance the system immunity against external interferences, integrated circuits with ultra-low noise current source for TMR biasing and low-noise variable gain amplifier are implemented. The integration procedures of advanced TMR sensors are explained in detail in [47]. Therefore, the miniaturised TMR-based sensing technologies make it possible to detect wearable and implantable MMG signals.

Here, we implemented a novel TMR sensor fabricated in International Iberian Nanotechnology Laboratory, operated at room temperature, to measure weak MMG signals [47]. Figure 4.6(d) shows the sensor image by a high-resolution microscope. There are 29 rows × 38 columns TMR elements in series and 1,102 in total, while the pads are 200 μm × 400 μm separated 250 μm. The enlarged images are shown in Figure 4.6(e) and (f), where each TMR element is 100 μm × 100 μm. The TMR stack consists of [5 Ta/25 CuN] × 6/5 Ta/5 Ru/20 IrMn/2 CoFe30/0.85 Ru/2.6 CoFe40B20/MgO [9 kΩ μm²]/2 CoFe40B20/0.21 Ta/4 NiFe/0.20 Ru/6 IrMn/2 Ru/5 Ta/10 Ru (unit: nm). With the bias current of 20 mA, the sensor offers 152% TMR ratio with a uniformity of 9% and an average R × A of 9 kΩ μm² with a 13% uniformity. For the full bridge setup, the measured voltage change per Oe per device is approximately 280 Ω μm²/Oe. Therefore, with 20 mA bias current and 1,102 devices, the sensitivity can reach approximately 0.617 V/Oe. It is worth mentioning that the sensor output is very close to zero with the absence of the external field and almost linear change around the zero point. Subsequently, an AFE circuit could help one to achieve the noise and offset cancellation.

ME sensors: A finite-size trilayer ME laminate structure is also designed, modelled and optimised using the FEM implemented in COMSOL. The main challenge of simulations is to accurately analyse the coupling of electric, magnetic and mechanical fields between MS and PE layers during the response of the ME laminate structures. To overcome this problem, these three coupled fields are computed in two steps. First, a static finite-element (FE) problem is analysed, allowing the calculation of the coefficients to build the constitutive law of the MS phase. The corresponding initial condition is without applied stress and the magnetic induction is produced as a result of the presence of the static magnetic field. The constant DC magnetic field driven by the coils should be accurately computed and the key variable is the uniform magnetic potential on the ME sensor. Second, a harmonic FE problem is discussed to solve the electric potential by applying a harmonic magnetic field at a resonance frequency.

Thin-film ME sensors are compatible with microelectronic processes without epoxy bonding, enabling devices with better consistency and smaller size. The compact FEM model is shown in Figure 4.5(h) where all layers are assumed internal-stress-free at zero applied fields. Here, we employed a laminated trilayer structure consisting of PE layer sandwiched between an MS layer and a silicon layer. The AlN and FeCoSiB are considered as PE and MS materials, respectively, while the poly-Si substrate is modelled as isotropic material. The overall computed displacements of the

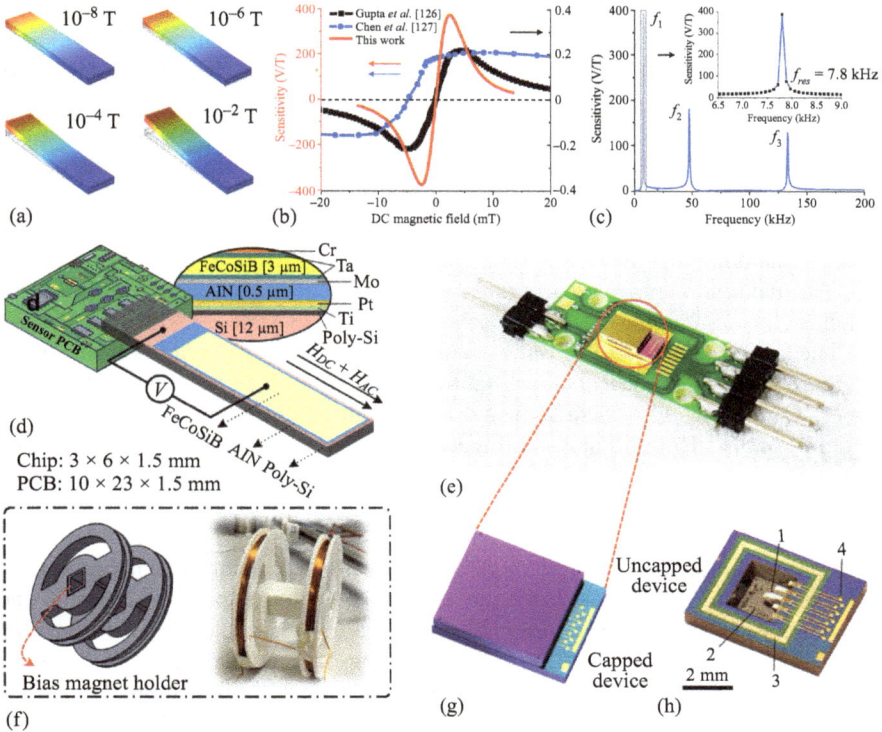

Figure 4.7 (a) The computed displacements of the ME sensor with magnitudes of an external magnetic field from 10^{-8} to 10^{-2} T; (b) the sensitivity of the longitudinal-transverse mode laminated ME sensor as a function of H_{DC}, compared to state-of-the-art experimental outcomes; (c) frequency dependence of sensitivity ($\mu_0 H_{bias} = 2$ mT); (d) schematic illustration of the fabricated ME sensor structure; (e) fabricated ME sensor (Fraunhofer Institute for Silicon Technology, Germany); (f) 3D printed circular Helmholtz coil where two magnets are put on both sides of the coil to provide constant dc bias field; photographs of a single sensor element: (g) capped device and (h) uncapped device with (1) ME cantilever, (2) etch groove, (3) bond frame and (4) bond pads

ME sensor from 10^{-8} to 10^{-2} T are demonstrated in Figure 4.7(a). For dynamic small AC magnetic field H_{AC}, the system can be solved linearly at a proper DC bias point. The calculated sensitivity of the longitudinal-transverse mode FeCoSiB/AlN/Poly-Si laminates as a function of the applied DC magnetic field, H_{DC}, is shown in Figure 4.7(b). In the beginning, the ME response curve is dramatically increased with weak magnetic fields, arriving the largest value, 382 V/T around 2 mT, which indicates that it reaches the maximum magnetostriction variation point. Subsequently, it is sharply decreased and finally vanished around 15 mT. The sensitivity curve shape matches very well with the fabrication results of the sandwiched composites [48]. Simulations predict higher sensitivities than observed in experiments [49,50], which we attribute to the nonideal magnetic properties in experimental MS layers.

Due to mechanical coupling between the PE and magnetic phases, the performance of the ME sensor is significantly enhanced if it is operated in a resonant state. Figure 4.7(c) shows the frequency response of the ME sensor at the bending mode through resolving eigenvalue problems and sweeping harmonic excitation frequencies. The maximum sensitivity occurs at the 7.8 kHz frequency of bending oscillations, which is almost 400 times higher than the low-frequency state.

The final proposed ME sensor structure considering its fabrication is illustrated in Figure 4.7(d). ME sensors were fabricated using surface micromachining processes. Cantilever chips were mounted on printed circuit boards (PCBs), and the top and bottom electrode connections were established manually. The fabrication details are demonstrated in [51]. Figure 4.7(e) shows the packaged and assembled device on a test board. The ME sensor consists of a thickness of 12 μm silicon cantilever, which is covered with a 0.5 μm thick PE aluminium nitride (AlN) on top. The third active layer is a 3 μm thick MS FeCoBSi top electrode with an area of $A = 2 \times 10^{-7}$ m^2. Additional layers are used for seeding, improving adhesion and insulation. A simple PCB (10 mm $\times$ 23 mm $\times$ 1.5 mm) is implemented with a chip dimension (3 mm $\times$ 6 mm $\times$ 1.5 mm). During sensor characterisation, magnets are utilised to provide a stable DC magnetic field which allows for operation of the ME at the optimum working point. We need another coil to produce a small AC field. Both magnetic fields are aligned parallel to the long axis of the ME sensor. Here, a 3D printed Helmholtz coil is designed and optimised, as shown in Figure 4.7(f). A pair of circular Helmholtz coils with the same direction of driven currents can generate a uniform region of the magnetic field. The ME sensor is then placed inside a magnetically shielded tube with a pair of magnets located on both sides of the coil but the radius of two circular coils and the distance between each other have the same value. Finally, Figure 4.7(g) and (h) gives detailed photographs of single encapsulated and non-encapsulated sensors with capped and uncapped devices [52].

A real-time readout system for these ME sensors has been proposed and implemented. The system architecture is illustrated in Figure 4.8(a), comprising sensors, AFE and digital back-end signal processing units. The stable power supplies are provided by voltage regulators. A power management unit with low-dropout regulators provides all required power supply voltages from a single 12 V battery. Finally, the signals are transmitted to a laptop and then extracted, classified and displayed in a graphical user interface based on LabVIEW. Based on the ME sensor principle, two types of amplifiers meet the requirements of the high impedance of the AFE, which are charge and voltage amplifiers. However, previous work has shown that the charge amplifier has a lower noise contribution than that of the voltage amplifier [53]. Therefore, a charge amplifier setup using an Analog Devices AD745 was chosen to measure the linear response of ME voltages.

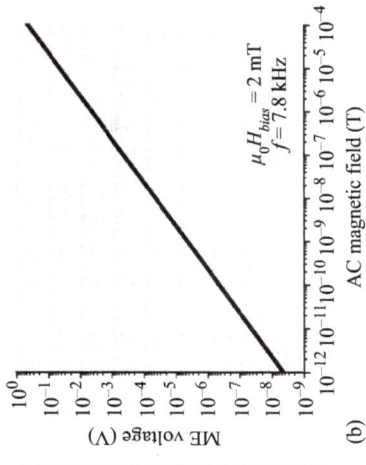

(a)

Equivalent circuit of ME sensor

Analog front-end

Other data acquisition architecture

A block diagram of a general processing chain for ME sensors in MMG measurements

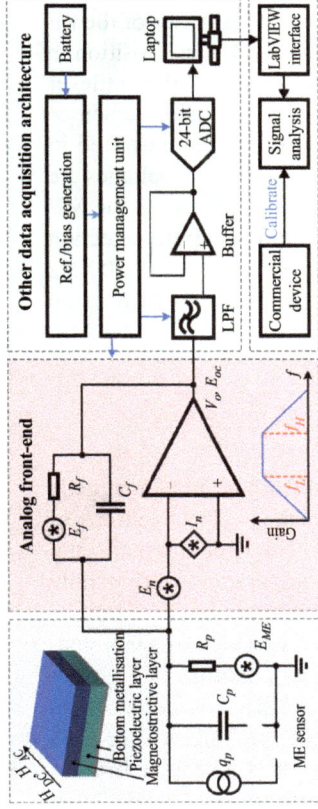

(c)

$\mu_0 H_{AC} = 1\ \mu T$
$\mu_0 H_{bias} = 1.6\ mT$

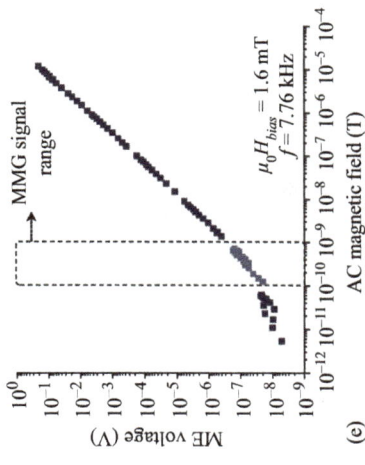

(b)

$\mu_0 H_{bias} = 2\ mT$
$f = 7.8\ kHz$

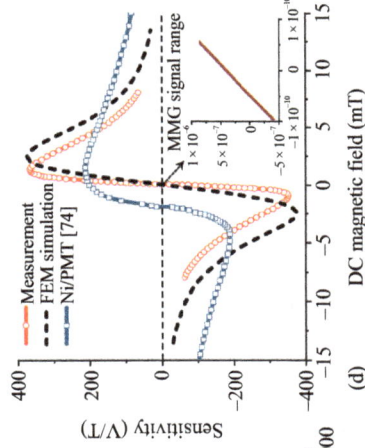

(d)

Measurement
FEM simulation
Ni/PMT [74]

MMG signal range

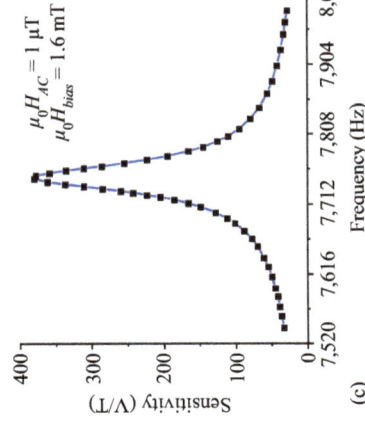

(e)

MMG signal range

$\mu_0 H_{bias} = 1.6\ mT$
$f = 7.76\ kHz$

Figure 4.8 (a) Overview of ME detection system. The recorded signals by the ME sensor are performed by digitally controlled analogue processing, which in general improves the readout of the sensor signals. The measured signals are passed to a digital signal enhancement stage before a detailed analysis can be performed; (b) ME voltage versus H_{AC} at the optimum working point ($H_{bias} = 2\ mT$ and $f = 7.8\ kHz$); (c) frequency dependence of sensitivity; (d) measured sensitivity as a function of the applied DC bias fields; (e) AC sensitivity and linearity

The FEM simulation results of induced voltages across the PE layer are shown in Figure 4.8(b), as an effective reference for the experiment. After an accurate sensor characterisation, the frequency dependence of the ME sensitivity is illustrated in Figure 4.8(c). It is measured with a stable bias DC magnetic field of $\mu_0 H_{bias} = 1.6$ mT and a low harmonic field of $\mu_0 H_{AC} = 1$ μT. A static sensitivity of 18 V/T is obtained using the quality factor, $Q = 2,217$, of the resonance curve when the ambient air pressure is zero. In addition, the ME response at a mechanical resonance state is observed. The maximum sensitivity is 378 V/T, obtained at the resonance frequency of 7.76 kHz. This is very consistent with the calculated value of 7.8 kHz in theory, calculated for the first resonance frequency [54]. Subsequently, the measured ME sensitivity in the response of external DC magnetic fields is compared with the simulation results and state-of-the-art fabrication outcome, Ni/PMT-based ME sensors [55]. At a resonance state, the sensitivity of up to 378 V/T is observed by applying an optimum DC bias field of $\mu_0 H_{bias} = 1.6$ mT, which is basically matched with the simulation results. The used poly-Si instead of SiO_2 as substrate increased the quality factor Q. Moreover, an optimisation of the thickness ratio between the MS and PE layers could lead to a higher α_{ME} [52]. In this case, the thicknesses of the PE and MS layers need to be carefully engineered to prevent a neutral plane position in one of the active layers [56]. A vacuum environment at a wafer level for ME cantilever encapsulation in this work also enhanced the Q, which further enlarged the sensor sensitivity [57]. The final AC sensitivity and linear response are demonstrated in Figure 4.8(e). At magnetic field values below 175 pT, the measured ME voltages are scattered due to a low SNR. However, as the field magnitude is increasing, the ME voltage exhibits a good linear response, which indicates its ultra-low field detection ability. To measure real MMG signals over a wide frequency band of 10–100 Hz without decreasing the noise level from the resonance state, the frequency conversion approach can be utilised.

4.3   MMG signal measurement

To reduce noise sources such as the acoustic noise and disturbances of magnetic and electric fields from the earth and surrounding equipment, characterisations of magnetic sensors were operated in a shielded environment. The experimental setup is shown in Figure 4.9(a). An active compensation technique is employed, mainly consisting of an active geomagnetic field cancellation box with an array of triaxial square Helmholtz coils and a reference magnetic device, THM1176 magnetometer from Metrolab Technology, Switzerland, in a triaxial configuration. The system is operated with the magnetic field compensation on three direction components (xyz) at the same time. In other words, $B_{(x,y,z)} = 0$. Thus, the measurement of each magnetic field component B_x, B_y and B_z of the geomagnetic field is cancelled. In addition, stainless steel tubes are put in the middle of the geomagnetic field cancellation box, forming 'double shielding'. The used equipment includes a triple-channel DC power supply (2230-30-1) from KEITHLEY Tektronix®, a stable DC power source (72-10500) from TENMA, a mixed domain oscilloscope (MDO3054), a digital

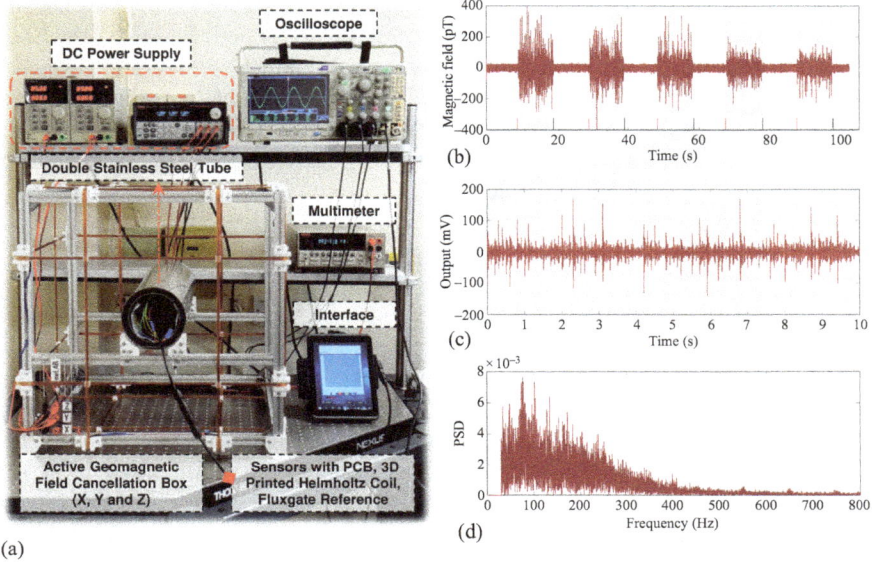

Figure 4.9 (a) Magnetic measurement setup with an active geomagnetic field cancellation box where double stainless steel tubes are in the middle; (b) measured MMG signals (100 s) from the proposed TMR system when the hand muscles were relaxed and tense, respectively; (c) MMG signals after a 20th-order bandpass Butterworth filter (30–300 Hz); (d) power spectrum from the tense hand muscles

precision multimeter (2000/E) from Tektronix. The results of the reference sensor, fluxgate (THM1176), is demonstrated in real time on the screen interface based on LabVIEW®.

The MMG demonstration takes TMR sensor as an example. Placing the TMR sensor array exactly on the skin of the abductor pollicis brevis hand muscle, the transverse component of the magnetic field can be accurately measured. The surface EMG signals were recorded at the same time as an effective reference. The 100-s MMG signals from the proposed TMR system were recorded and analysed to verify the whole process of muscle activities. Figure 4.9(b) shows a clear difference in time series between when the hand was tense and when the hand was relaxed. The first type is a time-domain with an amplitude of 200 pT, corresponding to periods when the hand is tense. This amplitude of the MMG signals corresponds to the accepted ideas about the magnetic field of skeletal muscles. The second type is a time-domain with an amplitude of 20–30 pT, corresponding to the lengths of time when the hand is relaxed. This amplitude is roughly equal to the amplitude of the noise activity records in a relaxed hand. Without filtering, the raw MMG signals from the tense muscles include wideband noise and movement artefacts. After using the 20th-order bandpass Butterworth filter of 30–300 Hz (Figure 4.9(c)), the signals not only became clearer but also confirmed that the positions of the peaks for both the MMG and EMG were almost the same. The approximate amplitude of 200 pT was observed, which is consistent with the reported value measured by SQUIDs. Finally, the MMG power spectrum is shown in Figure 4.9(d) with a wideband frequency range, in which the MMG signals of the tensed hand state is many times greater than noise. At frequencies from 30 to 300 Hz, the SNR is greater than 20.

4.4   Concluding remarks

MMG sensing is highly promising to extend the possibilities of EMG. Due to the low biomagnetic-field levels, it is a challenging task. Currently, new MMG sensor approaches are developed, which might enable implantable sensor modules completely encapsulated in a biocompatible material without any electrodes. The magnitude of the EMG signal is in the scale of millivolts and that for the MMG signal is in the scale of pT, depending upon different measurement conditions. The magnetic field of the Earth can reach values on the order of micro-tesla and the typical magnetic environmental noise can be on the order of 100 nT/Hz$^{1/2}$. However, the magnetic fields that are generated by the skeletal muscle are significantly smaller. In addition, it should be highlighted that the sensor interference (thermal and $1/f$ noises) largely degrades the response linearity and low-frequency detection ability in the TMR sensors. Various approaches have been studied to boost the SNR, including electromagnetic shielding techniques, reference channels and signal processing. Currently, there are no off-the-shelf solutions for the detection of MMG signals in non-magnetically shielded environments at room temperature. Essentially, the uniform background magnetic fields from the Earth would lead to saturating the sensor. Therefore, it would be a huge challenge to isolate the extremely weak biomagnetic components of the measured signals in the low-frequency domain (<500 Hz). A recent technique [58] to null the background static magnetic field in MEG consists of a shield to attenuate background noise from micro-tesla to nano-tesla. Then, a set of bi-planar electromagnetic coils generate nano-tesla fields equal and opposite to the remnant Earth's field, thereby cancelling it out. In addition, a proportional integral derivative algorithm was used to control the currents in the field-nulling coils. This allows the calculation of currents which generate fields that are equal and opposite to those measured by the reference array.

In the past, the measurements of the MMG signals were performed using SQUIDs with the detection limit of 3 fT/Hz$^{1/2}$ at 4 K. However, this technology is extremely expensive to both acquire and run and needs specialised facilities such as a shielded room and a cooling system. Moreover, SQUIDs detect the magnetic field at a short distance from the point of operation in the body. However, current human–machine interfacing concepts based on MMG rely greatly on the development of low-cost, flexible and miniaturised magnetic detectors. Flexible and miniaturised sensor structures show great potential to improve temporal and spatial resolutions, since the signal magnitude will be greater with the reduced distance between sensor and muscle tissue.

The magnitude of the MMG signal varies with the third power of the distance between the transducer and the current source. As a result, significant dimensional changes of the skeletal muscle during contraction or a movement of the human or the body part under investigation can affect the MMG signal, which can be troublesome. Consequently, all the human studies in vivo collected the MMG signal, while volunteers performed isometric contractions. Therefore, in order to avoid the effects of movement as much as possible, implantable MMG sensors would be more appropriate for human–machine interfacing, such as control of prosthetic limbs, to reduce the effect of muscle movement.

We described potential approaches for the next-generation recording of the MMG signals and discussed their benefits compared to conventional systems. The generation of the biomagnetic field by skeletal muscles was reviewed, compared with EMG and discussed in terms of the physical and mathematical relationships. In addition, the final characteristic properties of the main magnetic-sensor technologies for finding the optimal candidate of the MMG systems were provided. We advocated for the development of miniaturised magnetic sensors and the integration of MTJs into standard CMOS technology for MMG sensing. Then, we proposed several research strategies on how to fill the gap between the conventional and the next-generation MMG sensors that could achieve high-performance sensing. Moreover, we evaluated and discussed the challenges related to biomagnetic sensing such as nulling the magnetic field of the Earth. We provided a roadmap towards miniaturisation of magnetic sensors for low-field biomagnetic detection.

Future development of MR sensors will open new possibilities for the next generation of MMG systems. This includes the physical and functional properties of MR sensors and establishing new material systems. From the signal processing perspective, advanced data analysis techniques are highly required for cancelling the noise and offset at the sensors' output. We conclude that wearable and implantable MMG can soon become a promising and complementary approach for the measurement of muscle activity.

Acknowledgements

This work was supported by the Royal Society under grant RSG/R1/180269 and EP/R511705/1 from EPSRC, the United Kingdom. The work of KN is supported by grants EP/N023080/1 and EP/R004242/1 from EPSRC, the United Kingdom. Funding by the German Research Foundation (Deutsche Forschungsgemeinschaft DFG) through the Collaborative Research Center SFB 1261 'Magnetoelectric Sensors: From Composite Materials to Biomagnetic Diagnostics' is gratefully acknowledged.

References

[1]   Cohen D and Givler E. Magnetomyography: magnetic fields around the human body produced by skeletal muscles. Applied Physics Letters. 1972;21(3): 114–116.

[2]　Shin JOH. Clinical electromyography: nerve conduction studies. Baltimore: Williams and Wilkins; 1993.

[3]　Zuo S, Heidari H, Farina D, and Nazarpour K. Miniaturized magnetic sensors for implantable magnetomyography. Advanced Materials Technologies. 2020;2000185.

[4]　Grujić ZD, Koss PA, Bison G, and Weis A. A sensitive and accurate atomic magnetometer based on free spin precession. The European Physical Journal D. 2015;69(5):135.

[5]　Wijesinghe RS. Magnetic measurements of peripheral nerve function using a neuromagnetic current probe. Experimental Biology and Medicine. 2010;235(2):159–169.

[6]　Barbieri F, Trauchessec V, Caruso L, *et al.* Local recording of biological magnetic fields using giant magneto resistance-based micro-probes. Scientific Reports. 2016;6:39330.

[7]　Broser PJ, Knappe S, Kajal DS, *et al.* Optically pumped magnetometers for magneto-myography to study the innervation of the hand. IEEE Transactions on Neural Systems and Rehabilitation Engineering. 2018;26(11): 2226–2230.

[8]　Freitas PP, Ferreira R, and Cardoso S. Spintronic sensors. Proceedings of the IEEE. 2016;104(10):1894–1918.

[9]　Chen J, Lau Y, Coey JMD, Li M, and Wang J. High performance MgO-barrier magnetic tunnel junctions for flexible and wearable. Scientific Reports. 2017;7:42001.

[10]　Pannetier M, Fermon C, Le Goff G, Simola J, and Kerr E. Femtotesla magnetic field measurement with magnetoresistive sensors. Science. 2004; 304(5677):1648–1650.

[11]　Amaral J, Pinto V, Costa T, *et al.* Integration of TMR sensors in silicon microneedles for magnetic measurements of neurons. IEEE Transactions on Magnetics. 2013;49(7):3512–3515.

[12]　Amaral J, Gaspar J, Pinto V, *et al.* Measuring brain activity with magnetoresistive sensors integrated in micromachined probe needles. Applied Physics A: Materials Science and Processing. 2013;111(2):407–412.

[13]　Yamabe E, Nakamura T, Oshio K, Kikuchi Y, Ikegami H, and Toyama Y. Peripheral nerve injury: diagnosis with MR imaging of denervated skeletal muscle – experimental study in rats. Radiology. 2008;247(2):409–417.

[14]　Eswaran H, Govindan RB, Furdea A, Murphy P, Lowery CL, and Preissl HT. Extraction, quantification and characterization of uterine magnetomyographic activity – a proof of concept case study. European Journal of Obstetrics & Gynecology and Reproductive Biology. 2009;144:S96–S100.

[15]　Garcia MAC and Baffa O. Magnetic fields from skeletal muscles: a valuable physiological measurement? Frontiers in Physiology. 2015;6:1–4.

[16]　Farina D, Jiang N, Rehbaum H, *et al.* The extraction of neural information from the surface EMG for the control of upper-limb prostheses: emerging avenues and challenges. IEEE Transactions on Neural Systems and Rehabilitation Engineering. 2014;22(4):797–809.

[17] Krasoulis A, Vijayakumar S, and Nazarpour K. Multi-grip classification-based prosthesis control with two EMG-IMU sensors. IEEE Transactions on Neural Systems & Rehabilitation Engineering. 2020;28(2):508–518.

[18] Pistohl T, Cipriani C, Jackson A, and Nazarpour K. Abstract and proportional myoelectric control for multi-fingered hand prostheses. Annals of Biomedical Engineering. 2013;41(12):2687–2698.

[19] Antuvan CW, Ison M, and Artemiadis P. Embedded human control of robots using myoelectric interfaces. IEEE Transactions on Neural Systems and Rehabilitation Engineering. 2014;22(4):820–827.

[20] Dyson M, Barnes J, and Nazarpour K. Myoelectric control with abstract decoders. Journal of Neural Engineering. 2018;15(5):056003.

[21] Parker KK and Wikswo JP. A model of the magnetic fields created by single motor unit compound action potentials in skeletal muscle. IEEE Transactions on Biomedical Engineering. 1997;44(10):948–957.

[22] Heidari H, Zuo S, Krasoulis A, and Nazarpour K. CMOS Magnetic Sensors for Wearable Magnetomyography. In: 40th International Conference of the IEEE Engineering in Medicine and Biology Society; 2018. p. 2116–2119.

[23] Roth BJ and Wikswo JP. The magnetic field of a single axon. A comparison of theory and experiment. Biophysical Journal. 1985;48(1):93–109.

[24] Ganapathy N, Clark Jr JW, and Wilson OB. Extracellular potentials from skeletal muscle. Mathematical Biosciences. 1987;83(1):61–96.

[25] Hines ML and Carnevale NT. The NEURON simulation environment. Neural Computation. 1997;9(6):1179–1209.

[26] Malmivuo J and Plonsey R. Bioelectromagnetism: principles and applications of bioelectric and biomagnetic fields. New York, NY: Oxford University Press; 1995.

[27] Körber R, Storm J, Seton H, *et al.* SQUIDs in biomagnetism: a roadmap towards improved healthcare. Superconductor Science & Technology. 2016; 29(11):113001.

[28] Boto E, Meyer SS, Shah V, *et al.* A new generation of magnetoencephalography: room temperature measurements using optically-pumped magnetometers. NeuroImage. 2017;149:404–414.

[29] Karo H and Sasada I. Magnetocardiogram measured by fundamental mode orthogonal fluxgate array. Journal of Applied Physics. 2015;117(17): 17B322.

[30] Nakayama S and Uchiyama T. Real-time measurement of biomagnetic vector fields in functional syncytium using amorphous metal. Scientific Reports. 2015;5:1–9.

[31] Jogschies L, Klaas D, Kruppe R, *et al.* Recent developments of magnetoresistive sensors for industrial applications. Sensors. 2015;15(11):28665–28689.

[32] Freitas PP, Cardoso FA, Martins VC, *et al.* Spintronic platforms for biomedical applications. Lab on a Chip. 2012;12(3):546–557.

[33] Shen HM, Hu L, and Fu X. Integrated giant magnetoresistance technology for approachable weak biomagnetic signal detections. Sensors. 2018; 18(1):148.

[34]   Amaral J, Cardoso S, Freitas PP, and Sebastião AM. Toward a system to measure action potential on mice brain slices with local magnetoresistive probes. Journal of Applied Physics. 2011;109(7):07B308.

[35]   Pannetier-Lecoeur M, Fermon C, Dyvorne H, Jacquinot JF, Polovy H, and Walliang AL. Magnetoresistive-superconducting mixed sensors for biomagnetic applications. Journal of Magnetism and Magnetic Materials. 2010; 322(9–12):1647–1650.

[36]   Cubells-Beltrán MD, Reig C, Madrenas J, *et al.* Integration of GMR sensors with different technologies. Sensors. 2016;16(6):939.

[37]   Caruso L, Wunderle T, Lewis CM, *et al.* In-vivo magnetic recording of neuronal activity. Neuron. 2017;95(6):1283–1291.

[38]   Julliere M. Tunneling between ferromagnetic films. Physics Letters A. 1975; 54(3):225–226.

[39]   Nan CW, Li M, and Huang JH. Calculations of giant magnetoelectric effects in ferroic composites of rare-earth–iron alloys and ferroelectric polymers. Physical Review B. 2001;63(14):144415.

[40]   Röbisch V, Salzer S, Urs NO, *et al.* Pushing the detection limit of thin film magnetoelectric heterostructures. Journal of Materials Research. 2017;32(6):1009–1019.

[41]   Reermann J, Durdaut P, Salzer S, *et al.* Evaluation of magnetoelectric sensor systems for cardiological applications. Measurement. 2018;116:230–238.

[42]   Zuo S, Nazarpour K, and Heidari H. Device modeling of MgO-barrier tunneling magnetoresistors for hybrid spintronic-CMOS. IEEE Electron Device Letters. 2018;39(11):1784–1787.

[43]   Nabaei V, Chandrawati R, and Heidari H. Magnetic biosensors: modelling and simulation. Biosensors and Bioelectronics. 2017;103:69–86.

[44]   Paz E, Ferreira R, and Freitas PP. Linearization of magnetic sensors with a weakly pinned free-layer MTJ stack using a three-step annealing process. IEEE Transactions on Magnetics. 2016;52(7):1–4.

[45]   Zuo S, Fan H, Nazarpour K, and Heidari H. A CMOS Analog Front-End for Tunnelling Magnetoresistive Spintronic Sensing Systems. In: 2019 IEEE International Symposium on Circuits and Systems (ISCAS); 2019. p. 1–5.

[46]   Cardoso FA, Costa T, Germano J, *et al.* Integration of magnetoresistive biochips on a CMOS circuit. IEEE Transactions on Magnetics. 2012;48(11):3784–3787.

[47]   Zuo S, Nazarpour K, Böhnert T, Ferreira R, and Heidari H. Integrated Pico-Tesla Resolution Magnetoresistive Sensors for Miniaturised Magnetomyography. In: 42nd Annual International Conference of the IEEE Engineering in Medicine and Biology Society (EMBC); 2020. p. 1–5.

[48]   Dong S and Zhai J. Equivalent circuit method for static and dynamic analysis of magnetoelectric laminated composites. Chinese Science Bulletin. 2008;53(14):2113–2123.

[49]   Gupta R, Tomar M, Gupta V, *et al.* Giant magnetoelectric effect in PZT thin film deposited on nickel. Energy Harvesting and Systems. 2016;3(2):181–188.

[50]   Chen L and Wang Y. Enhanced magnetic field sensitivity in magnetoelectric composite based on positive magnetostrictive/negative magnetostrictive/

piezoelectric laminate heterostructure. IEEE Transactions on Magnetics. 2017;53(11):1–5.

[51]   Su J, Niekiel F, Fichtner S, *et al.* Frequency tunable resonant magnetoelectric sensors for the detection of weak magnetic field. Journal of Micromechanics and Microengineering. 2020.

[52]   Marauska S, Jahns R, Greve H, Quandt E, Knöchel R, and Wagner B. MEMS magnetic field sensor based on magnetoelectric composites. Journal of Micromechanics and Microengineering. 2012;22(6):65024.

[53]   Jahns R, Greve H, Woltermann E, Quandt E, and Knochel RH. Noise performance of magnetometers with resonant thin-film magnetoelectric sensors. IEEE Transactions on Instrumentation and Measurement. 2011;60(8):2995–3001.

[54]   Voiculescu I, Zaghloul ME, McGill RA, Houser EJ, and Fedder GK. Electrostatically actuated resonant microcantilever beam in CMOS technology for the detection of chemical weapons. IEEE Sensors Journal. 2005;5(4):641–647.

[55]   Zhou Y, Chul Yang S, Apo DJ, Maurya D, and Priya S. Tunable self-biased magnetoelectric response in homogenous laminates. Applied Physics Letters. 2012;101(23):232905.

[56]   Krantz MC, Gugat JL, and Gerken M. Resonant magnetoelectric response of composite cantilevers: theory of short vs. open circuit operation and layer sequence effects. AIP Advances. 2015;5(11):117230.

[57]   Lee B, Seok S, and Chun K. A study on wafer level vacuum packaging for MEMS devices. Journal of Micromechanics and Microengineering. 2003; 13(5):663.

[58]   Boto E, Holmes N, Leggett J, *et al.* Moving magnetoencephalography towards real-world applications with a wearable system. Nature. 2018;555(7698):657.

Chapter 5

Implantable technologies for closed-loop control of prosthesis

Ivo Strauss[1,2] and Silvestro Micera[1,2,3]

Nerves can be considered to be the information highways of our bodies. Having their own language they use the central nervous system (CNS) and peripheral nervous system (PNS) to manage our body. They immerge from the brain and distribute into the body branching off the more, the further you go. Electrical signals are transmitted to communicate between the CNS and the PNS.

In a broader spectrum, nerves are the only way to exchange information between our body and the environment. For example, we need them to control our hand movements, leg movements, eye movements, facial expressions, etc. This is crucial to take care of ourselves in daily life activities and to communicate with the outside world. With these functions missing, the quality of life drastically decreases. Spinal cord injury patients, for example, are not completely independent anymore. For example, to get from A to B, a person bound to the wheelchair will need a technically adapted car, public transport which is wheelchair-adapted and ramps or elevators to access every building. Depending on the country, this is not always the case.

For an upper limb amputee, for example, it takes usually much longer to get prepared in the morning. Taking a shower, shaving and dressing up is more time-consuming. Preparing food, opening bottles and cutting bread take a bigger effort. This also affects the way people interact with their social environment. And one of the most important factors: working nowadays almost always requires a PC. This becomes a severe problem, especially when it comes to writing and mouse-handling velocity. The effectiveness is drastically decreased and leads to the loss of job opportunities.

Neural interfaces make it possible to communicate with our nervous system. They can read (record) and thus manipulate and further create new inputs (stimulate). The challenge here is to develop a very selective, biocompatible and easy to implant electrode. The selectivity is important to be able to choose which part of the nerve branch should be programmed. The more specific you are, the more functionality and sensations can be given to the subjects.

[1]The BioRobotics Institute, Scuola Superiore Sant'Anna, Pisa, Italy
[2]Department of Excellence in Robotics & AI, The BioRobotics Institute, Scuola Superiore Sant'Anna, Pisa, Italy
[3]Bertarelli Foundation Chair in Translational NeuroEngineering, Centre for Neuroprosthetics and Institute of Bioengineering, École Polytechnique Fédérale de Lausanne (EPFL), Lausanne, Switzerland

Biocompatibility is an important aspect to provide the function of the implant and the safety of the implanted subjects. In a perfect condition, the implants should electrically work for a life time while not creating any harmful body reactions. In the real world, the body reacts with an acute inflammation and encapsulates foreign bodies (e.g. implants) over time. This influences the electrical properties in a negative way and leads to a reduced function or even a total failure. To reduce the foreign body reaction, and therefore reduce the possibility of implant failure, the implantation strategy should be chosen carefully. In general, as little damage as possible should be applied during the implantation. Finally the implantation time of the interface should be as short as possible to reduce the strain patients experience during and after the anesthesia.

To overcome these issues and optimize the quality of the patient's life, sensorized motor neuroprostheses can be used. In amputees, a stimulation of the nerves, proximally to the amputation level, is performed to provide sensory feedback of the missing limb. The electrical signal injected in the nervous tissue is sent to the brain, where, as a consequence, sensations can be perceived. In addition, the recording of motor neurons or surface EMG electrodes can be used to control robotic hands/legs prosthesis which is attached to the amputees stump. Closing the loop, it is possible for the amputee to use his prosthesis as if it would be his own hand. Movements of the artificial prosthesis are usually induced by myoelectric circuits controlling engines.

In para- or tetraplegic people, the situation is different. To overcome the missing connection between the CNS and PNS that is not given, a communication bridge has to be built. Patients' PNS is working but they cannot use it because the connection is interrupted (by, e.g., a spinal cord injury). This can be done implanting neural electrodes into the cortex registering the motor intentions of the subjects. As a consequence, motor neurons in the periphery can be stimulated to activate muscle contractions and move their upper limbs.

In this chapter, we will give an overview of the human nervous system, state-of-the-art neural interfaces and their application in upper limb amputees and paralyzed patients and how they can improve the quality of life.

5.1   Anatomy

5.1.1   Axons

Nerves provide the main pathway for the information exchange between the CNS and the periphery. This happens in the form of electrochemical impulse transmission along the axons. An axon is a structure formed by an axon and its supporting Schwann cells when found in the PNS.

Schwann cells are a particular type of glial cells of the PNS that support axons along their course. They can be myelinating or non-myelinating. Myelinating Schwann cells surround and wrap multiple times around the axon forming the myelin sheath. This sheath is an isolating lipidic coating that enhances the efficiency of nerve information propagation.

Table 5.1   Erlanger–Gasser classification of axon

Fiber type	d (μm)	V_c (m/s)	Myelinated
Aα	13–20	80–120	Yes
Aβ	6–12	33–75	Yes
Aγ	5–8	4–24	Yes
Aδ	1–5	3–30	Thin
B	1–5	3–15	Yes
C	0.2–1.5	0.5–2.0	No

As for mammals, approximately 75 percent of the cutaneous axons and 50 percent of the muscle axons (also motor fibers) are unmyelinated [1].

According to the direction of the conveyed information flow, fibers can be divided into afferent and efferent fibers: afferent fibers convey information from the PNS to the CNS, efferent fibers in the opposite direction.

According to the nature of the conveyed information flow, fibers can be divided into sensory fibers, carrying sensory information from the periphery to the CNS; motor fibers, controlling the contraction of skeletal muscles; and autonomic fibers, influencing the function of internal organs. In order to distinguish them from autonomic fibers, sensory and motor fibers are collectively referred to as somatic fibers. All sensory fibers are afferent, all motor fibers are efferent. An existing classification based on fiber conduction speed (V_c), which is strictly related to the diameter of the fiber (d), is called Erlanger–Gasser classification. In Table 5.1, we briefly outline the Erlanger–Gasser classification of axons [2].

5.1.2   From fibers to nerves

Axons (Figure 5.1) are organized into fascicles. The axons in a fascicle are immersed in a connective tissue called endoneurium. The endoneurium is organized in fine laminae around Schwann cells which produce the collagenous matrix in which few fibroblasts can be seen. The endoneurium is a permeable tissue that allows the passage of molecules still preventing the interference of the electrical activity of neighboring fibers. Each nerve fascicle is surrounded by multiple single-cell layers constituting the perineurium. Perineurial cells join in tight junctions forming a selectively permeable barrier. The perineurium allows some movement of axons within the fascicles; it concurrently maintains intrafascicular pressure and serves as a physical barrier against mechanical and chemical injuries.

In large-caliber nerves, such as the sciatic nerve, fascicles are surrounded by the inner epineurium. Two fascicles build up more complex structures called nerve branches. These structures do not intersect during the course of the nerve and will eventually separate into several branches. In the sciatic nerve, the peroneal and tibial nerves have such a role. They are surrounded by the outer epineurium and are further enclosed by the paraneurium that supports the nerve and connects it to the neighboring

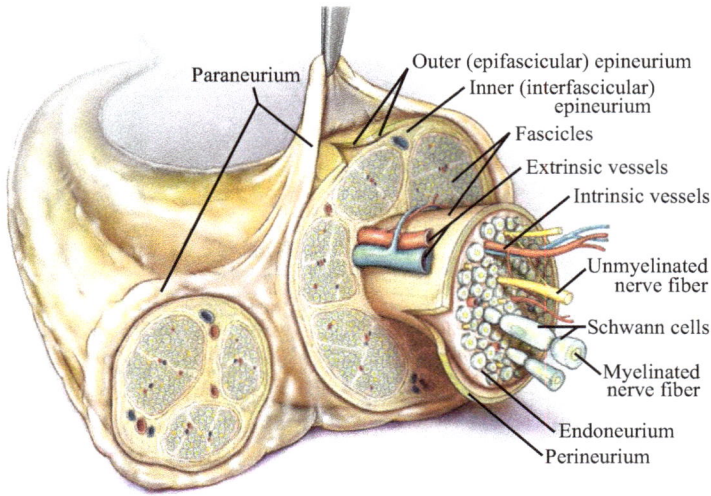

Figure 5.1   Illustration of large-caliber nerves such as the sciatic nerve. Two nerves are connected via the paraneurium. Inside each nerve, the epineurium holds together single fascicles, which contain the nerve axons [4]

structures. A pictorial representation of the sciatic nerve morphology can be seen in Figure 5.1 [3].

5.1.3   Central and peripheral nervous system

The basic function of the nervous systems is divided into three functional parts: the somatosensory, the motor and the autonomic nervous system. The somatosensory (also sensory) functions include the detection of stimuli, including taste, pain, touch, vision and hearing. Sensory (afferent neurons) transfer information in direction to the brain or spinal cord. So, the received information is then processed in the CNS (brain and spinal cord) to create a new output signal. The final response of this signal is determined by the processes happening in the CNS.

If touching a hot iron, for example, the polysynaptic reflex would cause a contraction of the biceps brachialis muscles to pull back the hand from the iron in a fast, involuntary movement. In this specific case, which is a somatic reflex, the information will not be passed to the brain but affect the muscle directly passing the so-called reflex arc in the spinal cord. When a reflex only includes two neurons (one sensory and one motor), it is called monosynaptic, whereas a reflex with more neurons is considered to be a polysynaptic reflex [5].

For example, autonomic functions are sleeping and waking cycle, language, thinking, reasoning, understanding, emotions and motivations [6].

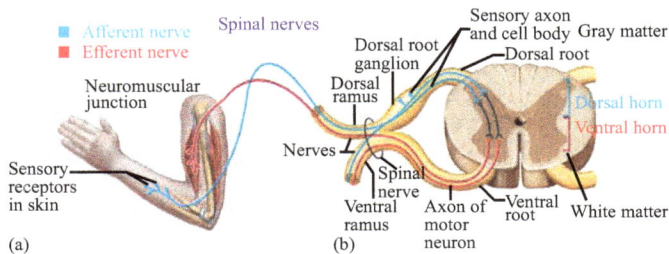

Figure 5.2   Function of the spinal nerves carrying motor, sensory and autonomic information. Location of the neuromuscular junction. Dorsal side is the back side and the other way around [7] (translated and adapted)

Our motor system carries information from the CNS (the brain and the spinal cord) to the effectors, that is, the muscles. The basic pathway is primary motor cortex, spinal cord, peripheral nerves and neuromuscular junctions, which you can partially see in Figure 5.2. The result will be a stimulation of the neuromuscular junction. In a functioning efferent system, cortical signals are sent to the periphery over an upper and a lower motor neuron.

The upper motor neuron tells the lower motor neuron when to start and when to stop activating the muscles. If a signal is created in the motor cortex (biochemically speaking, by the release of glutamate), a depolarization in the lower motor neuron is triggered. When the signal arrives at the gap between synapse and muscle cell, a neurotransmitter called acetylcholine is released causing the muscle cells to contract [5].

5.1.4   Electrical stimulation of neural tissue

The mechanism of stimulation of nerve cells relies on the change of the electrical potential of the nerve cells membrane. In the basic state, the membrane potential of a cell is approximately -70 mV [8]. The reason for this negative difference between the extra- and intracellular space is that usually more negative ions are at the inside than on the outside. Using ion-channels, the cell can transport and exchange these ions between the inside and outside. The transported ions are potassium (K+), sodium (Na+) and calcium ($-$Ca).

The channels can be activated by, e.g., electrical, mechanical and chemical factors. When, for example, mechanically touching a Pacini corpuscle (force sensor under the epiderma), Na+ channels will open, creating an inflow of ions leading to a positive change of the membrane potential. When a certain threshold of the resting potential is exceeded, the so-called action potential is created, traveling along the axons leading to, e.g., a muscular contraction. Figure 5.3 shows how the propagation of action potentials works. After the excitation of the presynaptic neuron, the action potential travels along the myelinated or non-myelinated axon.

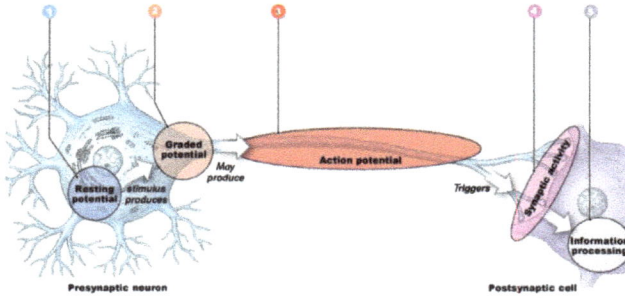

Figure 5.3   Signal propagation from presynaptic neuron to synapse. Depolarization happens in the soma and propagates over the myelinated axon to the synapse [9]

By changing the membrane potential of consecutively following nerve segments, the change of electrical potential continues until the end of the nerve cell (synapse). This process can literally be compared to a wave traveling along the axon. For the reason that fat insulates electricity, the myelin sheaths (see Figure 5.1) increase the transfer velocity of the action potentials [10].

Normally these signals are sent by the brain-coordinating body reactions and physical movements such as arm and leg movements, eye movements, bladder control and heartbeat frequency. For patients with a neural lesion or nerve amputation, it becomes difficult, or even impossible, to transmit these signals to the target destination. To overcome this lack of information, neural electrodes in combination with a neural prosthesis can be implanted.

5.1.4.1   Nerve anatomy and computational models

To make state-of-the-art neuroprosthetics work, it is essential to understand the fascicular anatomy of the nerves innervating the human hand. Information about the amount of afferent and efferent axons is essential to further develop the right intraneural electrode. Active stimulation sites have to be dimensioned in a way that they elicit the desired axonal population. Besides many others in 2017, a study on human cadavers which analyzed the fascicular distribution in the median, ulnar and radial nerves was performed [11–14]. They revealed important information such as fascicular count, the location of the fascicles and the fascicle diameters and distribution. Using this information, computational models as in Oddo's work from 2016 can be developed to predict mechanical, biological and electrical functionalities of neural electrodes [15].

5.2   Peripheral neural interfaces

Since almost 20 years, peripheral neural interfaces have been used to interface with the human nervous system. A broad community developed, and as a consequence the research on neural selectivity, biocompatibility and long-term stability increased. It became possible to read (record) and control (stimulate) the nervous system of living beings. With upcoming therapies (foot drop syndrome, depression, tremor, bladder dysfunction, amputation, etc.), different types of electrodes were developed to satisfy clinical needs.

One reason is that implantations in the periphery brings several advantages compared to CNS implants. First, it is much easier to get access to peripheral nervous structures, as there is no bone-like structure (e.g., scapula or vertebral column) protecting them. Further, the axons do not contain neural cell bodies, which prevents the CNS from taking damage, maintaining the whole processing power of the implanted individual. Also, infections are potentially less dangerous. Infection of an electrodes being implanted in the brain can therefore be much more life-threatening.

The challenge of peripheral implants is to get in contact with the right region of the nerve, i.e., fascicles, axon bundles or even singular axons. The ulnar and the median arm nerves, for example, are responsible for the sensory and motor innervation of the human palm. When providing sensory feedback, the goal would be to have one active site (AS) close to sensory-evoking axon bundles. By modifying the parameters of the injected current, it is then possible to modify the perceived sensations. The same accounts for recording in neural prosthesis. The closer and better dimensioned an AS is, the better the recording of such will be. Therefore, the control of the prosthesis will be better, and the patients will be more likely to enjoy their new device.

Selectivity in neural tissue

To give an example, 100 percent selective neural electrodes would be able to record or stimulate every single axon in the nerve separately. Hence, all afferent (sensation) as well as efferent (motor control) axons could be influenced in any constellation. Sensory feedback, for example, could be applied exactly where necessary. The patient could feel a sensation in the exact middle of his little finger when necessary. On the other hand, every motor intention of the user could be read from the single motor axons. Therefore, also the intensity of all the muscle contractions could be controlled.

Finally, three categories of neural interfaces showed to be most successful. There are epineural, intraneural and regenerative electrodes. Figure 5.4 gives an overview of the three categories. It is shown how the different electrode types interface with different nerve areas. The black portions represent the passive portion of the electrode. The yellow part shows where electrical current can be applied.

In the following chapter, a more detailed description of the state-of-the-art neural interfaces will be presented. We will describe conceptual approaches and discuss advantages and disadvantages of the currently existing electrodes.

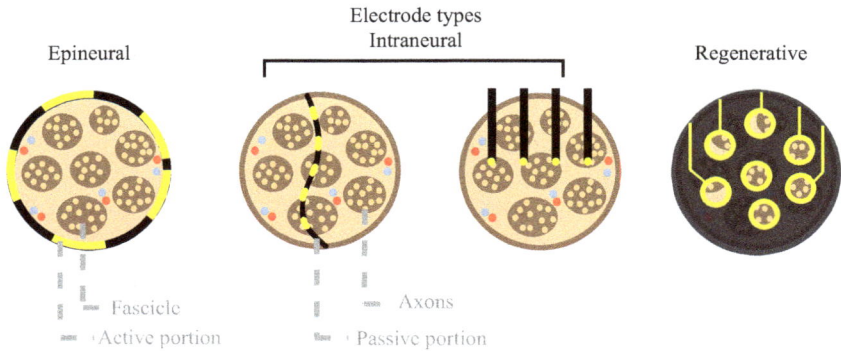

Figure 5.4   Active site locations and general shape of three different intraneural electrode types: epineural, intraneural and regenerative

5.2.1   Epineural electrodes

Epineural electrodes are placed around or on top of peripheral nerves. They have a round or rectangular structure which contains two or more electrical contacts. The insulating sheet is removed where the inner side of the electrode should be in contact with the nervous tissue. They can be used to record and stimulate nervous tissue.

Since they do not penetrate the nervous tissue, they are one of the least invasive electrodes. This brings the advantage that the implantation of such devices is quite straightforward. Also it permits the surgeons to perform corrections of the implant location if necessary. Furthermore, the stimulation and recording can be tested before the final fixation of the devices. Once in the right position, the epineural electrodes are usually sutured to the epineurium for fixation. The removal is less difficult than the implantation.

Regarding materials, mostly platinum or platinum–iridium contacts are used. Their electrical and mechanical properties make it possible to stimulate as well as record from nervous tissue. The active stimulation and recording sites are quite large compared to other electrode types. This does not make it necessary to apply superficial coatings to increase the stimulation and recording properties.

In 1961, Liberson *et al.* stimulate the peroneal nerve to reduce the side effects of the foot drop syndrome [16]. Later in the 1990s, epineural and cylindrical electrodes are gaining more and more interest. In 1994, Strege *et al.* apply stimulation for the relief of neuropathic pain [17]. In 1997, Chervin and Guilleminault [18] and Stanton-Hicks and Salamon [19] start to apply button-type (Button Cuff) electrodes to reduce traumatic injuries in long-term implants. In 1990, Napels *et al.* developed a helicoidal electrode (seen in Figure 5.5) for vagus nerve stimulation (VNS). It is adapting shape reduces the damage caused to the nerve. This electrode still finds application today.

Besides the helicoidal electrode, mostly multichannel cuffs are used in clinical and research applications of these days. Because of their reliability, they are easy to find and many companies offer them in many different variations.

In addition to the classical multichannel cuff, a more advanced cuff concept was developed by Choi in 2001 [20]. The flattening interface nerve electrode, short FINE, is made of the same materials as the classical fine. Like the name says, the FINE is flattening the nerve to get access to more fascicles. In classic FINEs, the electrical current does not necessarily penetrate the whole nerve [20,21].

After further developments, modifications and many years of experiments in animals, human cadavers and finally human amputees, the electrode has been accepted in the scientific community [22–26].

Very recently, a new approach was published by Cobo *et al.* [27] in which they presented a parylene C cuff that contained microfluidic channels. The channels were parallel to the nerve and made the axon fibers grow inside them. This could serve as the basis for a less invasive and much more selective approach.

5.2.2 Intrafascicular electrodes

Intrafascicular electrodes are electrodes that penetrate the nervous tissue in a transversal way and are in direct contact with the internal space of the nerves. In an optimal condition, the electrodes penetrate the fascicles and the ASs are close to the target axon bundles. Usually, the channel count is much higher compared to epineural electrodes. This drastically increases the fascicular selectivity and decreases the signal-to-noise-ratio of such electrodes. In addition, lower stimulation currents are necessary, since there is no epineurium protecting and electrically insulating the nerve. This is very useful for full implantable long-term implants which are battery dependent.

A side effect of higher selectivity is an increased damage of the implanted tissue. The consequence is a bigger inflammation of the tissue. As you can see in Figure 5.6, intrafascicular electrodes are in the middle field when it comes to selectivity versus invasiveness. With needle-guided implants such as the transversally inserted multichannel electrode (TIME) and the SELINE, it helps one to open the para- and epineurium to make sure that the electrodes are inserted inside the fascicles. This is why a very well-experienced neurosurgeon is necessary for such implants. This further reduces the total surgery time, of course, relieving the patients from the side effects of anesthesia.

Concerning the materials and technologies, many different approaches exist. One of the first generations is the longitudinal intrafascicular electrode, short LIFE. The LIFE concept was first introduced by Malagodi *et al.* in 1989 [28]. From there on the electrode developed very quickly and became well known in the scientific community. As principal investigator, Horch's group experimented with different materials such as Kevlar and polyimide wires as conduction support [29,30]. The final outcomes are two electrodes. The thin-film LIFE (tfLIFE) longitudinally inserted polyimide film with up to eight gold contacts [31]. And the distributed intrafascicular multielectrode and its newer version can have up to 15 contacts which are made with platinum/iridium wires and are connected to a fully implantable stimulator made by Cochlear Ltd., Sydney, Australia [32,33].

In 2010, the TIME, a longitudinally inserted multichannel electrode which is based on a polyimide film, was presented by Boretius *et al.* (see Figure 5.5). The basic

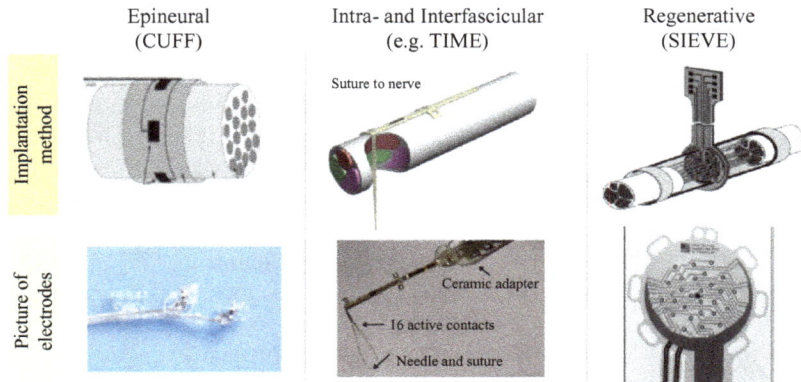

Figure 5.5   In yellow: illustration of implantation method of epineural, intraneural and regenerative electrodes. In green: the basic electrode schemes and actual pictures of the electrodes are shown [34,38]

concept allows the electrode to be inserted by folding a conductive 2D polyimide layer making a loop, which is connected to a micro suture. The micro-suture is fixed to a tungsten needle which is pulled through the peripheral nerve, inserting the TIME into the target tissue. In the last 10 years, intensive research improved the lead wire and their connection, the channel count and the coating strategies of the TIME [34–37]. The TIME can now hold up to 16 active stimulation and recording sites (plus 2 ground electrodes) and has an iridium-oxide coating to increase the maximum injectable charge [39].

A similar polyimide substrate electrode has been developed in 2011 by Micera's group in Pisa, Italy. A self-opening intraneural electrode (SELINE) should increase the stability and fixation, once the transversally inserted electrode is implanted [40–42]. The electrodes have been tested in in vivo experiments in rats [43]. Also in rabbits, optical nerve stimulating and recording of visually evoked cortical potentials has been performed [44].

Another approach which initially has been developed to be implanted as an intra-cortical (CNS) electrode has been transferred to the PNS. The Utah Slanted Electrode Array, short USEA, is made of high density silicon tips with a conducting center and tip. The electrode is inserted using a pressure gun and can contain up to 100 ASs. Chronic experiments in cats sciatic nerve showed that the electrode does not cause locomotion or behavioral deficits and can evoke motor potentials [45]. In 2011, it was possible to record neural signals for a period of 4 months [46]. After updating the electrode applying a better coating and improving the lead connections, in 2013, two tetraplegic patients managed to control a robotic arm, grasping and performing everyday tasks [47]. Very impressive progressions are still made today.

5.2.3   Regenerative electrodes

Regenerative electrodes can be applied when the implanted nerve has completely been transected or, for example, an organ is being transplanted. They are used to connect two nerve stumps which then regenerate through conducting holes which permit to register or stimulate the newly grown axons. They are considered to be one of the most selective types.

As the nerve has to be separated to implant a regenerative electrode, they are also considered to be one of the most invasive interfaces existing so far. To implant such devices, highly skilled and trained surgeons are required, as two nerve endings have to be sutured together, or at least to a supporting portion, which in the most banal case is a silicone tube. The fact that it takes time for the axons to regrow does not make regenerative electrodes suitable for acute experiments.

One of the first regenerative electrodes has been made by mechanically drilling holes into an epoxy modules [48]. Later, after microtechnology processes evolved, the supporting substrates became silicon substrates [49–52]. This made it possible to decrease the AS dimension and increase the AS number. As a result, it was possible to record neural activity of peripheral nerves [49,50,53].

However, this approach continued to create problems regarding the axonal regeneration and long-term stability which is why polyimide structures have been developed [54–56]. Polyimide showed to be much more suitable which is why this approach still is applied today.

5.2.4 Biocompatibility

Neural electrodes are made of conducting metals and supporting materials which are rigid and non-physiologic structures. Interfacing with neural tissue means to introduce a foreign, electrically conducting, rigid body in a naturally soft, wet and constantly changing environment. To make neural implants suitable for clinical applications, it is of profound importance to provide mechanical and electrical long-term functionality. In short, they should be biocompatible [57].

Biocompatibility

Is the ability of the device to perform its intended function, with the desired degree of incorporation in the host, without eliciting any undesirable local or systemic effects in that host.

One of the first reactions after implanting an electrode is the foreign body reaction, short FBR. The FBR is highly dependent on the tissue type and the geometry, stiffness, insertion strategy and also surface chemistry of the implanted electrode.

Similar to an injury, the body's alarm system immediately informs the CNS which, in turn, causes a coagulation cascade to control and fight the foreign body. Granulocytes, monocytes and macrophages migrate to the implantation site [58]. Around the implant, macrophages transform to foreign body giant cells (FBGCs) and the degradation of the implant material continues. FBGCs then activate fibroblasts which consequently lead to fibrotic tissue encapsulating the implant [59].

This encapsulation around the implanted electrodes increases the impedance and therefore decreases the maximal injectable charge of the electrode. Of course, also the capability of neural recording decreases. Signals are getting lower in amplitude and the chance to record single axon recordings decreases significantly.

To reduce the FBR as much as possible, animals and humans usually follow an anti-inflammatory therapy after the implantation. An additional solution is the active or chronic release of anti-inflammatory substances through the neural implant. Usually, they are applied locally or in the electrode integrated microchannels can be used to achieve this [60].

Further problems are the micro movements electrodes can experience. In acute as well as long-term implants, this can strongly influence the outcome of the final results. It becomes very difficult to compare the final results when recording locations change constantly [61].

5.2.5   Selectivity versus invasiveness

There is no existing device which provides the perfect selectivity and a low tissue invasiveness at the same time. Even if researchers are working on the miniaturization of existing electrodes to make them more invisible to the implanted tissue, there remains still is a trade-off. Sometimes, larger ASs are sufficient (e.g., foot drop syndrome) and sometimes very precise interfaces are necessary (neural recording for prosthesis control). Generally, all approaches aim on preserving the residual functions as well as possible and to harm the implanted tissue as less as possible.

In the neuroscientific community, there is a very distributed image available which shows the relation between the selectivity and the invasiveness of the before-mentioned electrode types. As many variations of electrode types exist, we adapted the relations to single electrodes (Button Cuff, Cuff, FINE, LIFE, TIME, USEA and SIEVE) to give a more specific overview (Figure 5.6).

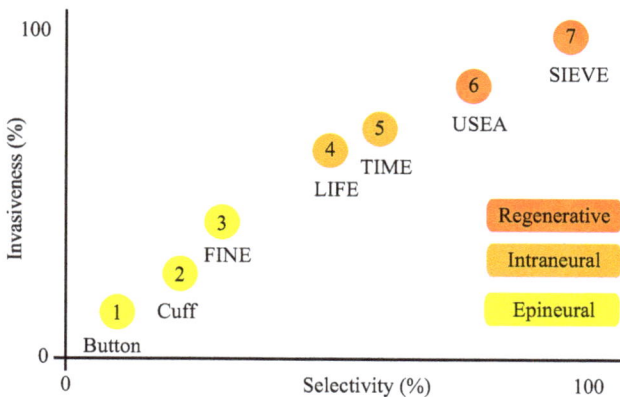

Figure 5.6   *Relation between invasiveness and selectivity between state-of-the-art electrodes to interface with peripheral nervous systems. The more invasive the electrode the more selective*

Of the implanted versions, one of the less invasive electrodes is the Button Cuff electrode. The fact that it is not surrounding the nervous tissue prevents any possible compression. The selectivity is due to a low amount of ASs, very low.

The multichannel cuff electrode is quite selective. It makes it possible to stimulate and record from different fascicles that are close to the epineurium of the nerve. The inside fascicles are hard to reach. Compared to the Button Cuff, the invasiveness is slightly increased because of the closed structure surrounding the nerve. The FINE is flattening the nerve thus getting a better access to the fascicles. The flattening process increases the invasiveness on the other hand.

The LIFE is similarly invasive to the TIME but has less and larger ASs and is therefore less selective. The difference is that the LIFE is inserted longitudinally and very close to the surface.

The TIME is quite invasive, since it penetrates through the nerve and its fascicles. Because of its high contact amount and the smaller ASs and their locations, it gets much more selective and can stimulate and record in terms of fascicles to axon groups.

The USEA is invasive because of its high count and density of electrodes. Being able to record from single units, the USEA has a very high selectivity. Following histological analysis, it does not penetrate the whole nerve and is therefore not very selective in respect to the whole nerve transection [12].

Regenerative electrodes have the highest selectivity but do need the nerve to be cut to be able to be implanted. This is considered to be the highest level of invasiveness.

5.3 Application fields of neural interfaces

5.3.1 Upper limb prosthesis control

The loss of a lower or upper limb significantly affects people's lives. Upper limb amputees mostly suffer from phantom limb pain and a lack of sensory input when using artificial prosthesis, which does not provide the dexterous of a real hand. For example, they cannot use their hand without looking at it. This reduces the utility and often lets the patients unsatisfied which can further lead to complete abandonment [62,63].

Restoring the functionality of a missing limb using a robotic prosthesis, or via predicting the kinetics of the movement in general, e.g., [64], it needs to solve two main issues: decoding motor intentions of the subject and restoring the afferent information flow from sensor readings to the brain. Having somatotopic sensations coherent with the interaction with the environment is fundamental for fostering the phenomena of embodiment, in which the subject includes the prosthesis into its mental body image, proving a complete acceptance. Here, the quality of the sensation plays an important role. Therefore, a strong community of researches started to study in this direction.

5.3.1.1 Sensory feedback and prosthesis control

So far many approaches have been made to provide sensory feedback in amputees (Figure 5.7). In 2012, Horch *et al.* implanted two upper limb amputees with LIFEs to provide object discrimination capabilities. One of the subjects was able to perceive

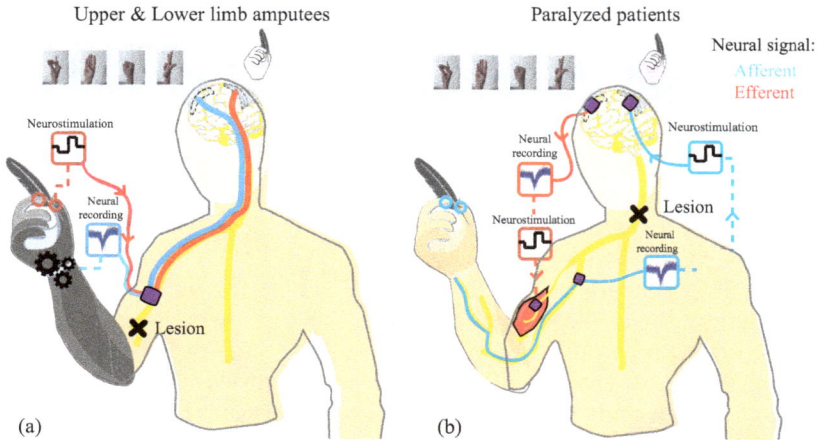

Figure 5.7   Basic principles of bidirectional systems: (a) trans-radial amputee with a bidirectional prosthesis providing sensory feedback by intraneural stimulation. The prosthesis actuators can be controlled by motor intentions and neural recordings; (b) motor and sensory rehabilitation approach for paralyzed people

indentation of two fingers and a proprioceptive movement, making a fist and feeling the fingers curling inward. Standard EMG surface electrodes were used to control the prosthesis hands opening and closing [65].

Tan *et al.* implanted two subjects with cuffs and FINEs successfully providing patients with chronically stable sensations such as touch and light moving touch. Phantom limb pain could be eliminated in both the subjects. The subjects could perform grasping experiments for more than 48 months. For myoelectric prosthesis control classical superficial dry EMG electrodes from Otto Bock were used to perform opening and closing of the hand [25,26].

Ortiz-Catalan *et al.* published an osseo-integrated interface in 2014. This novel approach made it possible to first provide sensory feedback in a completely integrated closed-loop system for 1 year. One spiral cuff was used to stimulate the ulnar nerve. The most evoked sensation was mostly a tingling. Phantom limb pain could be reduced by 40 percent. For EMG recording, two bipolar and four monopolar epimyseal electrodes were used to control the prosthetic hand and elbow. They made it possible to reduce the force being necessary to activate the prosthesis actuators [66].

With standard surface EMG electrodes, the threshold of the muscle activation has to be over 60 percent. With the epimyseal electrodes 15 percent is sufficient, thus less effort is required. Finally, it was possible for the patient to perform hand opening and closing, wrist pronation and supination, wrist flexion and extension and elbow flexion and extension with a final average accuracy of 95.4 percent [66].

Davis *et al.* implanted two patients with 96 channel USEA electrodes for 30 days. Intraneural peripheral stimulation evoked very concentrated sensations on different parts of the fingers (median nerve stimulation) and on fingers and palm during ulnar nerve, stimulation. Subjects mostly perceived vibration and tingling. Subject two added that the vibration and tingling sensation was mostly perceived as painful. Recording neural activity from the median or ulnar nerve, they managed to online decode the flexion movement of two fingers in each subject [67].

In 2017, Wendelken *et al.* again implanted two human subjects with two USEA electrodes each (one in the ulnar, one in the median nerve) for 4–5 weeks. The patients were able to reach a sensory feedback of 26 percent proprioception, 32 percent tingling, 25 percent vibration and 17 percent pressure. Regarding the movements, five degrees of freedom (DOF) could be distinguished in one subject. They were using a virtual hand to display the online decoded movement. After 13 days, the neural recording capacities decreased continuously [68].

In 2010, Rossini *et al.* implanted one subject with four tfLIFEs for a period of 4 weeks. Two electrodes were implanted in the median, and two in the ulnar nerve. The subject reported touch and tingling sensations during intraneural stimulation. Sensations were reported at the base of the index and middle finger and the center palm when stimulating the median nerve. For ulnar nerve stimulation a radiating sensation (wrist to finger) was reported. They recorded neural signals and applied a wavelet de-noising for spike-sorting purposes. The identified waveforms were used to train a support vector machine classifier to decode motor intentions and translate them into prosthesis movements [69].

Raspopovic *et al.* [70] continued with the implantation of one subject with four TIME electrodes implanted in median and ulnar nerve. During intraneural stimulation, a touch sensation was reported on the index and thumb (median nerve stimulation), and on the little finger (ulnar nerve stimulation). For the control, five surface EMG signals were used. For classification, a multilayer perception network has been applied. It was possible to perform palm grasp, pinch grasp, ulnar grasp, open hand and rest movement. Finally, it was possible to use the sensory information perceived by the subject to fine control three different force levels in real time.

A very recent publication by Petrini *et al.* [71] extended the previous investigations on sensory feedback using four TIMEs in each subject. Three subjects were implanted for a period of 6 months each providing sensory feedback. A very intensive mapping procedure was performed to evaluate the sensations perceived by the subjects. The most perceived sensations were vibration in subjects one and three and electricity subject two. In average, all subjects could perceive five different sensation levels. Blindfolded, force control, pick and lift and a virtual eggs test have been performed, to promote and further understand the embodiment of prosthesis when receiving intraneural stimulation [72].

Recovering motor functions in paralyzed subjects addresses a different problem. The limb is functional, but the control signal coming from the brain is missing because of an interruption in the CNS (e.g., spinal cord). The optimal strategy would be to consider the paralyzed limbs as a bio-robotic device being equipped with biological actuators and sensors. Actuating them using the signals which are derived from the

CNS could therefore considered to be a suitable solution. Passively or actively moving paralyzed limbs on the other hand is considered to be a therapy and has been proven to enhance residual functions significantly. Further it prevents articulation problems such as arthritis and promotes the function of the vascular system. On the other side, the control of devices becomes crucial for tetraplegic and locked in syndrome patients to be able to communicate with the outside world. The perfect combination would be a system where the patients could use their residual sensory signals to control their extremities, creating an artificial gap over the spinal lesion and their missing functions.

5.3.1.2   Functional motor neurostimulation

The application of specific currents to motor neurons has the effect of generating contractions in the connected muscles. This technique is defined as functional electrical stimulation (FES) or functional neuromuscular stimulation. The force applied by stimulated muscles can be modulated acting on stimulation parameters, such as the amplitude, pulse width and the frequency. In this way, it is possible to control them as biological actuators, with a known stimulation to force relationship.

Stimulating devices are usually used in open-loop configuration, where the user relies only on vision and other indirect means such as sensory feedback. One of the first attempts to design a portable FES system was done by Buckett in 1988. A total of 22 patients tested the device assistance in two types of grasping motions over 5 years; 11 of them used that on a daily basis. The results were successful, proving that FES is a suitable method for restoring hand functionality [73].

In complex gestures such as reaching, grasping and walking, multiple muscles are activated with patterns that are repeatable; these patterns are defined synergies.

Functional motor neurostimulation has been proven to be effective in restoring normal gait movements in people with moderate hemiplegia and spasticity, correcting, for example, the foot drop syndrome. The "Actigait" system from Ottobock is an example of a commercial device providing this solution.

FES was applied with success on subjects with thoracic level spinal cord injuries. For example, by Triolo's work in 2012, helping subjects with sit-to-stand transitions and to stand in a stable way without help. Further, patients could use their upper limbs increasing their autonomy in daily activities [74].

Complex tasks such as walking or grasping need plenty of controlled DOF, usually far more than the motor intentions extracted for the user. This limit can be overcome decoding only high-level directives from the user (walk forward, stop, grab, etc.) and let a low-level controller deal with fine control of all the muscles. Such controllers would need sensors to close the feedback loop and control the muscles autonomously.

The first motor stimulation systems were developed to be directly controlled by the users. Buttons or levers were used to manually control gestures. Closed-loop control then minimized the overstimulation of the muscles allowing them to apply only the minimum force needed to accomplish tasks.

The sensorization of lower and upper limbs is not an easy task. Particularly with limbs, sensors can influence residual functionalities in a negative way. Therefore, miniaturization plays an important role. An interesting approach is the exploitation of the sensors already present inside the skin. Signals recorded of neural activity could be used in a control loop.

One of the first attempts in this direction has been implemented by Haugland, after some studies with animals in 1994, to prove that slip events can be deduced from neural activity of afferent fibers [75]. In 1999, a complete closed loop implanted on a quadriplegic subject worked as expected, reducing to the minimum the needed force for grasping and automatically adjusting the stimulation to prevent the object from slipping [76].

In 2004, Inmann further improved these results, optimizing ENG decoding and successfully testing the system performances in daily living activities [77].

Low-level closed-loop control has a further advantage. It ensures high-speed responses to the user, enabling the immediate correction steps in lower limb. This reduces falling risk and increases grip force precision.

5.3.1.3   Read sensory information from PNS

Cuff electrodes are the most used devices to long-term interface with the PNS. In addition to their low invasiveness, they are appreciated for their mechanical and electrical stability. Due to their design, the signal recorded by cuff electrodes is a weighted sum of the signals traveling along the implanted nerve, with a higher presence of superficial fibers, multichannel electrodes try to overcome this limit enabling higher selectivity.

In 1994, experiments were performed where a cuff electrode recorded neural signals to control an event-driven gripping reflex mechanism. The cuff was implanted on a cat's tibial nerve while stroking over the cat's paw [75].

More advanced machine-learning techniques such as fuzzy systems and neural networks have been proven to successfully include less complex variables, such as joint angles for a general higher precision [78,79].

Information about slip events and applied force have been extracted by Haugland in 1994 from ENG recordings of afferent sensory fibers in humans. In this way, it was possible to implement a closed-loop controller to avoid the object to slip after the user completed its volitional grasping motion. The neural signal from the sural nerve was proven to be informative about heel strike events, providing a more reliable feedback than sensors placed on the body or sensorized insoles [80]. Haugland and Sinkjaer in 1995 designed a portable FES device able to restore normal gait movements thanks to information coming from ENG recordings [81].

Technology innovations in electrode design and advanced signal processing techniques promise to improve results in this field even further. As a significant example, in 2019 Song tested with success in animals a cuff electrode capable of both stimulating and recording in closed loop, paving the way for compact and more functional implanted systems [82].

5.4   Outlook

5.4.1   *Amputees of the future—bidirectional prosthesis*

We now know that research will make it possible in the near future to provide upper and lower limb amputees with prosthesis devices that are voluntarily controllable and can provide sensory feedback to the users. There are many possibilities and we do not yet know which system will be the most efficient and most convenient one.

Fact is that concerning upper and lower limb amputees, the final goal is to have a myoelectric, prosthetic arm or leg that can record efferent signals coming from the brain to control a prosthetic device. To do so, a neural implant with high selectivity, high biocompatible and an easy and straightforward implantation strategy is provided.

Furthermore, a lightweight prosthetic arm or leg with sufficient sensory input is necessary. The perfect solution would be a lightweight device that can be adapted to the original hand or leg weight of the user to provide also ergonomic stability. Of course, a sufficient sensorization and motor control of the used device is not less important.

Regarding para- and tetraplegic patients, a different approach has to be made. The target goal will be to restore their missing functions as good as possible by providing them with the possibility to control their limbs using peripheral FES. The power to control their nonfunctioning limbs and legs will optimally come from a brain–computer interface.

By simply thinking about a task such as grasping an object, pulling a handle, pressing a button, walking, sitting down, etc., the brain–computer interface will record the motor intention to then activate the target muscle regions. Of course, a very sophisticated stimulation pattern will be necessary to achieve such complicated tasks in a stable manner. In the future, this will significantly increase the therapy value and make it possible for the patients to regain a significant amount of independence. One of the most difficult tasks in the future will be to develop a closed-loop system that combines all the state-of-the-art technologies, is lightweight, is portable, is energy-efficient and most importantly is easy to use. Systems that are too complicated for the user will not be accepted in long-term.

An example is driving a car. People turn on the car and drive away using the steering wheel, gear box and pedals. If they would need to open the hood, connect the battery, control the brake fluid, etc. before they can go, then car driving probably would not have been that successful.

5.4.2 The bioelectronic human

Compared to pharmaceutical therapies, bioelectronic medicine (see Figure 5.8) offers the advantage to provide pain relief, heart rate modulation, depression relief, etc. without the side effects pharmaceuticals can cause.

In the United States, the fourth leading cause of death is drug side effects, which results in 100,000 deaths each year [83]. Despite computational strategies and in vitro and in vivo tests, and technologies that have been developed to test drugs before they are released to the market, there is no guarantee that there will be no other side effects.

In depression, patients' electrical stimulation could prevent abuse and dependency. The CNS or peripheral neural stimulation would reduce or completely relieve the patients from chronic pain. There would be no longer the risk of side effects, or the risks that after the therapy are addicted to the drug.

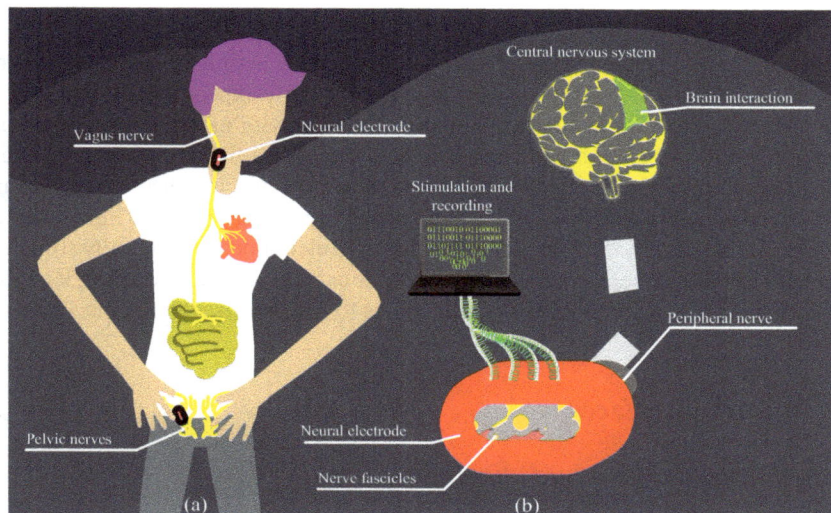

Figure 5.8   *Principles and examples of bioelectronic medicine: (a) vagus nerve stimulation influences the autonomic nervous system. Pelvic and sacral nerve stimulation can control incontinence and erectile functions; (b) neural electrodes are used to stimulate and record from nerves*

VNS, for example, is already proved to be a very potential neurostimulation therapy. The vagus nerve is the connection between the CNS and the autonomic nervous system, controlling heart rate, bladder function, digestive tract, liver, respiration and spleen. Recently, VNS therapies treating depression and drug-resistant epilepsy received the US Food and Drug Administration approval that opens the gate to other clinical trial applications such as heart rate control after transplantation, inflammation control of sepsis, lung injury, rheumatoid arthritis, diabetes and others [84].

Another successful example is the stimulation of sacral nerves to restore bladder functions and fecal incontinence in people with paraplegia [85].

TENS (transcutaneous electrical neural stimulation) for pain relief to reduce menstrual pain is another example of applied electro cuticle applications [86]. In general, 60–70 percent of women experience mild pain and 10–15 percent suffer from severe pain affecting their quality of life. In the United States, for example, the most occurring cause for school and working hour absence is dysmenorrhea [87]. Also here the main approaches to pain treatment are usually pharmacological solutions [88].

Also, the restoration of erectile dysfunctions in spinal cord injury patients or elderly people is upcoming. Even here the standard solutions are pharmaceutical such as Viagra, Levitra, Staxyn, etc., severely straining the vascular system with every intake. Again, neural stimulation provides a solution.

5.4.2.1   The challenges

It has been shown that neural stimulation has an effect on peripheral and the CNS and that we can use these signal highways to alter our daily life experience. But up to now, most of the electro cuticle interfaces do not stimulate with naturalistic patterns but they simply block or alternate the signal flow in the nerves. To be able to completely control the effects and side effects of electro cuticle therapies, it is therefore necessary to get a deeper understanding of the stimulation patterns we have to send into the tissue to get the desired target reaction. For example, VNS electrodes superficially stimulate more than 100,000 fibers, where each of them innervates a different target location. Simulation and model approaches could help us to resolve these problems.

5.5   Future interfaces

5.5.1   Focused ultrasound stimulation

The most common applications of ultrasound (US) are the monitoring of fetal developments and the observation of cardiac abnormalities. In the last decades, the capabilities of a new approach, the focused ultrasound (FUS), have shown to be stimulating and/or inhibiting neural activity. As a consequence, several approaches have been made, testing FUS also in the PNS. Starting with the single stimulation of myelinated in vitro axons by Mihran 1990, work developed quickly to more sophisticated approaches [89].

In the 1990s, the stimulation of skin, soft tissue, fingers, upper forearm and hand nerve endings was performed [90–92]. Further in vivo setups such as the one developed by Juan in 2013 revolutionized the US stimulation of humans. With different frequencies they were distally stimulating the vagus nerve of rats and recording the resulting nerve activity (proximally) with cuff electrodes [93]. A clear inhibition of the vagus nerve activity could be shown.

Nonetheless, there are some critical conclusions to make [94]. So far, first, there is no study that proves that the direct activation of peripheral nerves was possible by US stimulation alone. Second, there are suggestions that nerve blocks are caused only by the thermal effect that high-intensity US stimulation creates [95–97].

There are studies in mice and humans (median nerve stimulation) which show that US stimulation can enhance the conduction velocity of $A\alpha$- and C-type axons in in vivo experiments [98,99]. This lets us conclude that the blocking and enhancing of neural signals using US stimulation is applicable, but further studies will need to be conducted to fully understand the effects of US stimulation in peripheral nerves.

5.5.1.1   Optogenetics stimulation

One of the main reasons to use optical stimulation in nervous tissue is the low amount of energy it takes, the cell-type-specific stimulation and the low threshold activation of, for example, motor neurons. Given these properties, it would be possible to substitute FES when aiding patients with physical impairments. Examples are degenerative diseases that cause nonfunctioning or weakness in lower or upper limbs.

The main issues with the usually applied superficial FES are that large motor axons are activated before the small ones [100–102]. This is not physiological and permits further only a very coarse control of the muscles. Furthermore, FES causes the activation of unwanted receptors such as nociceptors (causing pain) and cutaneous mechanoreceptors [103]. Finally, this leads to a fast fatigue of the muscles, leaving the patients unsatisfied [103].

A very recently published article from Srinivasan *et al.* in 2018 presented a closed-loop optogenetic stimulation system which made it possible to control flexion and extension of several rats hind limb stimulating the tibial and peroneal nerve [104]. They showed that similar to Ortiz-Catalan's study of 2014, it was possible to reduce the muscle fatigue compared to FES [66].

In the same year, another article in *Nature Biomedical Engineering* has been published by Maimon [105]. Here, optogenetic stimulation was used to target the lower limb effectors relying on the retrograde transfection to restrict axonal opsin expression to the desired fiber targets.

A different paper published in Scientific Reports by Song *et al.* in 2018 showed the successful application of an optical cuff electrode simultaneously monitoring and stimulating in mice sciatic nerve [106].

Optogenetics is a very impressive approach but there are still some issues to resolve. A light source usually spreads in every direction and which is why it is difficult to target precise stimulation locations. Further disadvantages are a possible heating of the target tissue and a restriction in stimulation depth [107,108].

References

[1] Ochoa J. Recognition of unmyelinated fiber disease: morphologic criteria. Muscle & Nerve. 1978;1(5):375–387.

[2] Gasser HS. The classification of nerve fibers. Ohio Journal of Science. 1941;41:145–159.

[3] Reina MA, Sala-Blanch X, Arriazu R, and Machés F. Microscopic Morphology and Ultrastructure of Human Peripheral Nerves. In: Tubbs RS, Rizk E, Shoja MM, Loukas M, Barbaro N, and Spinner RJ, editors. Nerves and Nerve Injuries. London: Academic Press; 2015. p. 91–106.

[4] Gentry J. Peripheral Nerve Anatomy; 2019. Available from: https://www.medillsb.com/illustration_image_details.aspx?AID=3366&IID=132650.

[5] Biologie Anatomie Physiologie; 2019. Available from: https://shop.elsevier.de/biologie-anatomie-physiologie-9783437268038.html.

[6] Schmidt RF. Integrative Functions of the Central Nervous System. In: Schmidt RF, Thews G, editors. Human Physiology. Berlin, Heidelberg: Springer Berlin Heidelberg; 1989. p. 124–165.

[7] Watson C, Paxinos G, and Kayalioglu G. The Spinal Cord: A Christopher and Dana Reeve Foundation Text and Atlas. 1st ed. London: Academic Press; 2008.

[8]   A quantitative description of membrane current and its application to conduction and excitation in nerve. Accessed July 2019. Available from: https://www.ncbi.nlm.nih.gov/pmc/articles/PMC1392413/.

[9]   Biomedical Engineering Theory and Practice – Wikibooks, open books for an open world. Accessed July 2019. Available from: https://en.wikibooks.org/wiki/Biomedical_Engineering_Theory_And_Practice.

[10]   Fehlings MG, Vaccaro AR, and Boakye M. Essentials of Spinal Cord Injury: Basic Research to Clinical Practice. New York, NY: Thieme; 2012.

[11]   Brill NA and Tyler DJ. Quantification of human upper extremity nerves and fascicular anatomy. Muscle & Nerve. 2017;56(3):463–471.

[12]   Christensen MB, Wark HAC, and Hutchinson DT. A histological analysis of human median and ulnar nerves following implantation of Utah slanted electrode arrays. Biomaterials. 2016;77:235–242.

[13]   Slutsky DJ. Sensory Nerve Transfers in the Hand. In: The Art of Microsurgical Hand Reconstruction. 2013th ed. Thieme Verlag; 2013.

[14]   Delgado-Martínez I, Badia J, Pascual-Font A, Rodríguez-Baeza A, and Navarro X. Fascicular Topography of the Human Median Nerve for Neuroprosthetic Surgery. Frontiers Neuroscience; 2016. p. 10.

[15]   Oddo CM, Raspopovic S, and Artoni F. Intraneural stimulation elicits discrimination of textural features by artificial fingertip in intact and amputee humans. eLife. 2016;5:09148.

[16]   Liberson WT, Holmquest HJ, Scot D, and Dow M. Functional electrotherapy: stimulation of the peroneal nerve synchronized with the swing phase of the gait of hemiplegic patients. Archives of Physical Medicine and Rehabilitation. 1961;42:101–105.

[17]   Strege DW, Cooney WP, Wood MB, Johnson SJ, and Metcalf BJ. Chronic peripheral nerve pain treated with direct electrical nerve stimulation. The Journal of Hand Surgery. 1994;19(6):931–939.

[18]   Chervin RD and Guilleminault C. Diaphragm pacing for respiratory insufficiency. Journal of Clinical Neurophysiology. 1997;14(5):369–377.

[19]   Stanton-Hicks M and Salamon J. Stimulation of the central and peripheral nervous system for the control of pain. Journal of Clinical Neurophysiology. 1997;14(1):46–62.

[20]   Choi AQ, Cavanaugh JK, and Durand DM. Selectivity of multiple-contact nerve cuff electrodes: a simulation analysis. IEEE Transactions on Biomedical Engineering. 2001;48(2):165–172.

[21]   Schiefer MA, Triolo RJ, and Tyler DJ. A model of selective activation of the femoral nerve with a flat interface nerve electrode for a lower extremity neuroprosthesis. IEEE Transactions on Neural Systems and Rehabilitation Engineering. 2008;16(2):195–204.

[22]   Freeberg MJ, Stone MA, Triolo RJ, and Tyler DJ. The design of and chronic tissue response to a composite nerve electrode with patterned stiffness. Journal of Neural Engineering. 2017;14(3):036022.

[23]   Dweiri YM, Stone MA, Tyler DJ, McCallum GA, and Durand DM. Fabrication of high contact-density, flat-interface nerve electrodes for recording

and stimulation applications. Journal of Visualized Experiments. 2016:116. Available from: https://europepmc.org/backend/ptpmcrender.fcgi?accid=PM C5092158&blobtype=pdf.

[24] Polasek KH, Hoyen HA, Keith MW, Kirsch RF, and Tyler DJ. Stimulation stability and selectivity of chronically implanted multicontact nerve cuff electrodes in the human upper extremity. IEEE Transactions on Neural Systems and Rehabilitation Engineering. 2009;17(5):428–437.

[25] Tan DW, Schiefer MA, Keith MW, Anderson JR, Tyler J, and Tyler DJ. A neural interface provides long-term stable natural touch perception. Science Translational Medicine. 2014;6(257):257ra138.

[26] Tan DW, Schiefer MA, Keith MW, Anderson JR, and Tyler DJ. Stability and selectivity of a chronic, multi-contact cuff electrode for sensory stimulation in human amputees. Journal of Neural Engineering. 2015;12(2): 026002.

[27] Cobo AM, Larson CE, and Scholten K. Parylene-based cuff electrode with integrated microfluidics for peripheral nerve recording, stimulation, and drug delivery. Journal of Microelectromechanical Systems. 2019;28(1):36–49.

[28] Malagodi MS, Horch KW, and Schoenberg AA. An intrafascicular electrode for recording of action potentials in peripheral nerves. Annals of Biomedical Engineering. 1989;17(4):397–410.

[29] Lawrence SM, Dhillon GS, and Horch KW. Fabrication and characteristics of an implantable, polymer-based, intrafascicular electrode. Journal of Neuroscience Methods. 2003;131(1–2):9–26.

[30] McNaughton TG and Horch KW. Metallized polymer fibers as leadwires and intrafascicular microelectrodes. Journal of Neuroscience Methods. 1996;70(1):103–110.

[31] Yoshida K, Hennings K, and Kammer S. Acute Performance of the Thin-Film Longitudinal Intra-Fascicular Electrode. In: 2006 The First IEEE/RAS-EMBS International Conference on Biomedical Robotics and Biomechatronics (BioRob); 2006. p. 296–300.

[32] Thota AK, Kuntaegowdanahalli S, and Starosciak AK. A system and method to interface with multiple groups of axons in several fascicles of peripheral nerves. Journal of Neuroscience Methods. 2015;244:78–84.

[33] Pena AE, Kuntaegowdanahalli SS, Abbas JJ, Patrick J, Horch KW, and Jung R. Mechanical fatigue resistance of an implantable branched lead system for a distributed set of longitudinal intrafascicular electrodes. Journal of Neural Engineering. 2017;14(6):066014.

[34] Boretius T, Yoshida K, and Badia J. A Transverse Intrafascicular Multichannel Electrode (TIME) to Treat Phantom Limb Pain – Towards Human Clinical Trials. In: 2012 4th IEEE RAS EMBS International Conference on Biomedical Robotics and Biomechatronics (BioRob); 2012. p. 282–287.

[35] Čvančara P, Lauser S, Rudmann L, and Stieglitz T. Investigations on Different Epoxies for Electrical Insulation of Microflex Structures. In: 2016 38th Annual International Conference of the IEEE Engineering in Medicine and Biology Society (EMBC); 2016. p. 1963–1966.

[36] Stieglitz T, Boretius T, Čvančara P, *et al.* On Biocompatibility and Stability of Transversal Intrafascicular Multichannel Electrodes—TIME. In: Ibáñez J, González-Vargas J, Azorín JM, Akay M, and Pons JL, editors. Converging Clinical and Engineering Research on Neurorehabilitation II. Cham: Springer International Publishing; 2017. p. 731–735.

[37] Krähenbühl S, Čvančara P, and Stieglitz T. Return of the cadaver: Key role of anatomic dissection for plastic surgery resident training. Medicine (Baltimore). 2017;96:e7528.

[38] Navarro X, Krueger TB, Lago N, Micera S, Stieglitz T, and Dario P. A critical review of interfaces with the peripheral nervous system for the control of neuroprostheses and hybrid bionic systems. Journal of Peripheral Nervous System. 2005;10(3):229–258.

[39] Čvančara P, Boretius T, López-Álvarez VM, *et al.* Stability of thin-film metallization in flexible stimulation electrodes: analysis and improvement of in vivo performance. bioRxiv; 2019. Available from: https://www.biorxiv.org/content/early/2019/05/22/644914.

[40] Cutrone A, Sergi PN, Bossi S, and Micera S. Modelization of a self-opening peripheral neural interface: a feasibility study. Medical Engineering & Physics. 2011;33(10):1254–1261.

[41] Cutrone A, Del Valle J, and Santos D. A three-dimensional self-opening intraneural peripheral interface (SELINE). Journal of Neural Engineering. 2015;12(1):016016.

[42] Rehberger F, Stieglitz T, and Eickenscheidt M. Micro-Folded 3D Neural Electrodes Fully Integrated in Polyimide. In: 2018 40th Annual International Conference of the IEEE Engineering in Medicine and Biology Society (EMBC); 2018. p. 4587–4590.

[43] Wurth SM, Capogrosso M, Raspopovic S, *et al.* Long-term usability and bio-integration of polyimide-based intra-neural stimulating electrodes. Biomaterials. 2017;122:114–129.

[44] Gaillet V, Cutrone A, Vagni P, *et al.* Optic nerve intraneural stimulation allows selective visual cortex activation. bioRxiv; 2018. Available from: https://www.biorxiv.org/content/early/2018/05/07/311035.

[45] Petrini FM, Valle G, Strauss I, *et al.* Six–month assessment of a hand prosthesis with intraneural tactile feedback. Annals of Neurology, 2019;85:137–154.

[46] Clark GA, Ledbetter NM, Warren DJ, and Harrison RR. Recording Sensory and Motor Information from Peripheral Nerves with Utah Slanted Electrode Arrays. In: 2011 Annual International Conference of the IEEE Engineering in Medicine and Biology Society; 2011. p. 4641–4644.

[47] Hochberg LR, Bacher D, Jarosiewicz B, *et al.* Reach and grasp by people with tetraplegia using a neurally controlled robotic arm. Nature. 2012;485(7398):372–375.

[48] Mannard A, Stein RB, and Charles D. Regeneration electrode units: implants for recording from single peripheral nerve fibers in freely moving animals. Science. 1974;183(4124):547–549.

[49] Kovacs GTA, Storment CW, Halks-Miller M, *et al.* Silicon-substrate microelectrode arrays for parallel recording of neural activity in peripheral and cranial nerves. IEEE Transactions on Biomedical Engineering. 1994;41(6):567–577.

[50] Navarro X, Calvet S, Butí M, *et al.* Peripheral nerve regeneration through microelectrode arrays based on silicon technology. Restorative Neurology and Neuroscience. 1996;9:151–160.

[51] Akin T, Najafi K, Smoke RH, and Bradley RM. A micromachined silicon sieve electrode for nerve regeneration applications. IEEE Transactions on Biomedical Engineering. 1994;41(4):305–313.

[52] Wallman L, Zhang Y, Laurell T, and Danielsen N. The geometric design of micromachined silicon sieve electrodes influences functional nerve regeneration. Biomaterials. 2001;22(10):1187–1193.

[53] Mensinger AF, Anderson DJ, and Buchko CJ. Chronic recording of regenerating VIIIth nerve axons with a sieve electrode. Journal of Neurophysiology. 2000;83(1):611–615.

[54] Navarro X, Calvet S, and Rodríguez FJ. Stimulation and recording from regenerated peripheral nerves through polyimide sieve electrodes. Journal of Peripheral Nervous System. 1998;3(2):91–101.

[55] Ceballos D, Valero-Cabré A, Valderrama E, Schüttler M, Stieglitz T, and Navarro X. Morphologic and functional evaluation of peripheral nerve fibers regenerated through polyimide sieve electrodes over long-term implantation. Journal of Biomedical Materials Research. 2002;60(4):517–528.

[56] Lago N, Ceballos D, Rodríguez FJ, Stieglitz T, and Navarro X. Long term assessment of axonal regeneration through polyimide regenerative electrodes to interface the peripheral nerve. Biomaterials. 2005;26(14):2021–2031.

[57] Williams DF. On the mechanisms of biocompatibility. Biomaterials. 2008;29(20):2941–2953.

[58] McNally AK and Anderson JM. Beta1 and beta2 integrins mediate adhesion during macrophage fusion and multinucleated foreign body giant cell formation. American Journal of Pathology. 2002;160(2):621–630.

[59] Anderson JM, Rodriguez A, and Chang DT. Foreign body reaction to biomaterials. Seminars in Immunology. 2008;20(2):86–100.

[60] Eming SA, Krieg T, and Davidson JM. Inflammation in wound repair: molecular and cellular mechanisms. Journal of Investigative Dermatology. 2007;127(3):514–525.

[61] Gilletti A and Muthuswamy J. Brain micromotion around implants in the rodent somatosensory cortex. Journal of Neural Engineering. 2006;3(3): 189–195.

[62] Biddiss EA and Chau TT. Upper limb prosthesis use and abandonment: a survey of the last 25 years. Prosthetics and Orthotics International. 2007;31(3):236–257.

[63] Wijk U and Carlsson I. Forearm amputees' views of prosthesis use and sensory feedback. Journal of Hand Therapy. 2015;28(3):269–278.

[64]   Nazarpour K, Ethier C, Paninski L, Rebesco J, Miall RC, and Miller L. EMG prediction from motor cortical recordings via a non-negative point process filter. IEEE Transactions Biomedical Engineering. 2012;59(7): 1829–1838.

[65]   Horch K, Meek S, Taylor TG, and Hutchinson DT. Object discrimination with an artificial hand using electrical stimulation of peripheral tactile and proprioceptive pathways with intrafascicular electrodes . IEEE Transactions on Neural Systems and Rehabilitation Engineering. 2011;19(5): 483–489.

[66]   Ortiz-Catalan M, Håkansson B, and Brånemark R. An osseointegrated human-machine gateway for long-term sensory feedback and motor control of artificial limb. Science Translational Medicine. 2014;6(257):257re6.

[67]   Davis TS, Wark HAC, and Hutchinson DT. Restoring motor control and sensory feedback in people with upper extremity amputations using arrays of 96 microelectrodes implanted in the median and ulnar nerves. Journal of Neural Engineering. 2016;13(3):036001.

[68]   Wendelken S, Page DM, and Davis T. Restoration of motor control and proprioceptive and cutaneous sensation in humans with prior upper-limb amputation via multiple Utah Slanted Electrode Arrays (USEAs) implanted in residual peripheral arm nerves. Journal of NeuroEngineering and Rehabilitation. 2017;14(1):121.

[69]   Rossini PM, Micera S, and Benvenuto A. Double nerve intraneural interface implant on a human amputee for robotic hand control. Clinical Neurophysiology. 2010;121(5):777–783.

[70]   Raspopovic S, Capogrosso M, and Petrini FM. Restoring natural sensory feedback in real-time bidirectional hand prostheses. Science Translational Medicine. 2014;6:222ra19.

[71]   Petrini FM, Valle G, and Strauss I. Six-month assessment of a hand prosthesis with intraneural tactile feedback. Annals of Neurology. 2019;85(1): 137–154.

[72]   Rognini G, Petrini FM, and Raspopovic S. Multisensory bionic limb to achieve prosthesis embodiment and reduce distorted phantom limb perceptions. Journal of Neurology, Neurosurgery and Psychiatry. 2018;90(7):318570.

[73]   Buckett JR, Peckham PH, Thrope GB, Braswell SD, and Keith MW. A flexible, portable system for neuromuscular stimulation in the paralyzed upper extremity. IEEE Transactions on Biomedical Engineering. 1988;35(11): 897–904.

[74]   Triolo RJ, Bailey SN, and Miller ME. Longitudinal performance of a surgically implanted neuroprosthesis for lower-extremity exercise standing, and transfers after spinal cord injury. Archives of Physical Medicine and Rehabilitation. 2012;93(5):896–904.

[75]   Haugland MK and Hoffer JA. Slip information provided by nerve cuff signals: application in closed-loop control of functional electrical stimulation. IEEE Transactions on Rehabilitation Engineering. 1994;2(1):29–36.

[76] Haugland M, Lickel A, Haase J, and Sinkjaer T. Control of FES thumb force using slip information obtained from the cutaneous electroneurogram in quadriplegic man. IEEE Transactions on Rehabilitation Engineering. 1999;7(2):215–227.

[77] Inmann A and Haugland M. Implementation of natural sensory feedback in a portable control system for a hand grasp neuroprosthesis. Medical Engineering & Physics. 2004;26(6):449–458.

[78] Cavallaro E, Micera S, Dario P, Jensen W, and Sinkjaer T. On the inter-subject generalization ability in extracting kinematic information from afferent nervous signals. IEEE Transactions on Biomedical Engineering. 2003;50(9):1063–1073.

[79] Song K, Chu J, Park SE, Hwang D, and Youn I. Ankle-angle estimation from blind source separated afferent activity in the sciatic nerve for closed-loop functional neuromuscular stimulation system. IEEE Transactions on Biomedical Engineering. 2017;64(4):834–843.

[80] Haugland MK, Hoffer JA, and Sinkjaer T. Skin contact force information in sensory nerve signals recorded by implanted cuff electrodes. IEEE Transactions on Rehabilitation Engineering. 1994;2(1):18–28.

[81] Haugland MK and Sinkjaer T. Cutaneous whole nerve recordings used for correction of footdrop in hemiplegic man. IEEE Transactions on Rehabilitation Engineering. 1995;3(4):307–317.

[82] Song KI, Park SE, Hwang D, and Youn I. Compact neural interface using a single multichannel cuff electrode for a functional neuromuscular stimulation system. Annals of Biomedical Engineering. 2019;47(3): 754–766.

[83] Giacomini KM, Krauss RM, Roden DM, Eichelbaum M, Hayden MR, and Nakamura Y. When good drugs go bad. Nature. 2007;446:975–977.

[84] Johnson RL and Wilson CG. A review of vagus nerve stimulation as a therapeutic intervention. Journal of Inflammation Research. 2018;11: 203–213.

[85] Al-Sannan B, Banakhar M, and Hassouna MM. The role of sacral nerve stimulation in female pelvic floor disorders. Current Obstetrics and Gynecology Reports. 2013;2(3):159–168.

[86] Tugay N, Akbayrak T, and Demirtürk F. Effectiveness of Transcutaneous Electrical Nerve Stimulation and Interferential Current in Primary Dysmenorrhea. Pain Medicine. 2007;8(4):295–300.

[87] Hillen TI, Grbavac SL, Johnston PJ, Straton JA, and Keogh JM. Primary dysmenorrhea in young Western Australian women: prevalence, impact, and knowledge of treatment. Journal of Adolescent Health. 1999;25(1):40–45.

[88] Coco AS. Primary dysmenorrhea. American Family Physician. 1999;60(2): 489–496.

[89] Mihran RT, Barnes FS, and Wachtel H. Transient modification of nerve excitability in vitro by single ultrasound pulses. Biomedical Sciences Instrumentation. 1990;26:235–246.

[90]   Gavrilov LR, Gersuni GV, Ilyinski OB, Tsirulnikov EM, and Shchekanov EE. A study of reception with the use of focused ultrasound I. Effects on the skin and deep receptor structures in man. Brain Research. 1977;135(2):265–277.

[91]   Ithel Davies I, Gavrilov LR, and Tsirulnikov EM. Application of focused ultrasound for research on pain. Pain. 1996;67(1):17–27.

[92]   Dalecki D, Child SZ, Raeman CH, and Carstensen EL. Tactile perception of ultrasound. The Journal of the Acoustical Society of America. 1995;97:3165–3170.

[93]   Mihran RT, Barnes FS, and Wachtel H. Temporally-specific modification of myelinated axon excitability in vitro following a single ultrasound pulse. Ultrasound in Medicine & Biology. 1990;16(3):297–309.

[94]   Feng B, Chen L, and Ilham SJ. A review on ultrasonic neuromodulation of the peripheral nervous system: enhanced or suppressed activities? Applied Sciences. 2019;9(8):1673.

[95]   Colucci V, Strichartz G, Jolesz F, Vykhodtseva N, and Hynynen K. Focused ultrasound effects on nerve action potential in vitro. Ultrasound in Medicine & Biology. 2009;35(10):1737–1747.

[96]   Foley JL, Little JW, and Vaezy S. Image-guided high-intensity focused ultrasound for conduction block of peripheral nerves. Annals of Biomedical Engineering. 2007;35(1):109–119.

[97]   Foley JL, Little JW, and Vaezy S. Effects of high-intensity focused ultrasound on nerve conduction. Muscle & Nerve. 2008;37(2):241–250.

[98]   Jawad Ilham S, Chen L, Guo T, Emadi S, Hoshino K, and Feng B. In vitro single-unit recordings reveal increased peripheral nerve conduction velocity by focused pulsed ultrasound. Biomedical Physics & Engineering Express. 2018;4(4):045004.

[99]   Moore JH, Gieck JH, Saliba EN, Perrin DH, Ball DW, and McCue FC. The biophysical effects of ultrasound on median nerve distal latencies. Electromyography and Clinical Neurophysiology. 2000;40(3):169–180.

[100]   Llewellyn ME, Thompson KR, Deisseroth K, and Delp SL. Orderly recruitment of motor units under optical control in vivo. Nature Medicine. 2010;16(10):1161–1165.

[101]   Mendell LM. The size principle: a rule describing the recruitment of motoneurons. Journal of Neurophysiology. 2005;93(6):3024–3026.

[102]   Malmivuo J and Plonsey R. Bioelectromagnetism: Principles and Applications of Bioelectric and Biomagnetic Fields. New York, NY: Oxford University Press; 1995.

[103]   Currier D and Mann R. Pain complaint: comparison of electrical stimulation with conventional isometric exercise. Journal of Orthopaedic & Sports Physical Therapy. 1984;5(6):318–323.

[104]   Srinivasan SS, Maimon BE, Diaz M, Song H, and Herr HM. Closed-loop functional optogenetic stimulation. Nature Communications. 2018;9(1):5303.

[105]   Maimon BE, Sparks K, Srinivasan S, Zorzos AN, and Herr HM. Spectrally distinct channelrhodopsins for two-colour optogenetic peripheral nerve stimulation. Nature Biomedical Engineering. 2018;2(7):485.

[106] Song KI, Park SE, Lee S, Kim H, Lee SH, and Youn I. Compact optical nerve cuff electrode for simultaneous neural activity monitoring and optogenetic stimulation of peripheral nerves. Scientific Reports. 2018;8(1):15630.

[107] Wells J, Kao C, and Konrad P. Biophysical mechanisms of transient optical stimulation of peripheral nerve. Journal of Biophysics. 2007;93(7):2567–2580.

[108] Thompson AC, Wade SA, Brown WGA, and Stoddart PR. Modeling of light absorption in tissue during infrared neural stimulation. Journal of Biomedical Optics. 2012;17(7):075002.

Chapter 6
Direct neural control of prostheses via nerve implants

Benjamin William Metcalfe[1], Dingguo Zhang[1] and Thomas dos Santos Nielsen[2]

The primary goal of direct neural control is to provide a seamless interface to the body's own control and feedback systems. In the case of an upper limb amputation, such an interface would ideally enable a direct mapping of motor commands and sensory feedback to and from a prosthesis and the undamaged portion of the nervous system. In theory, this interface could be constructed in such a way that control of the prosthesis was *transparent* to the user, feeling as close as possible to the original limb. This idealised paradigm would require no training or learning on the part of the user or the prosthesis. To provide this level of natural control, an interface is required between the peripheral nervous system (PNS) and the prosthesis. In practice, of course, no such ideal interface exists. However, recent developments in electrode design, biocompatible materials and signal processing are paving the way for the emergence of superior interfaces in the future.

Fundamentally, a peripheral nerve interface must achieve two goals: recording the motor commands sent from the brain from the severed proximal nerve stump and the stimulation of the same proximal stumps to elicit sensory feedback. These signals form the basic feedforward and feedback paths of a closed-loop prosthetic. The two goals must be achieved using an electrode structure that is implanted on or in the nerve. Thus, the electrodes should be capable of interfacing bidirectionally to specific motor and sensory pathways in a manner that is minimally invasive, stable in time and with the best possible biocompatibility. A further, more speculative, goal of such interfaces is the reduction of phantom limb pain that can occur when sensory signals are restored to the residual nerves.

The main aim of this chapter is to review the technology and strategy currently in development for creating bidirectional peripheral nerve interfaces within the upper limb.

At present, the most common approach for control of upper limb prostheses is to place surface electrodes onto the skin over intact muscle in the proximal limb stump. The amputee can then selectively activate these muscles and the resulting electrical

[1]Department of Electronic and Electrical Engineering, University of Bath, Bath, UK
[2]Department of Health Science and Technology, University of Aalborg, Aalborg, Denmark

signals (the electromyogram, EMG) may be recorded and translated to perform pre-defined movements. This approach is advantageous in that surface electrodes are non-invasive and well tolerated. The EMG signals tend to be quite large, thus easy to record, and new signal processing techniques are continually advancing the capabilities of this approach. In general, however, this approach has been limited to one or two degrees of movement in the prosthesis. It is difficult to extract detailed movement intentions and, depending on the residual muscles available, the amputee will likely have to spend significant time learning new and unfamiliar muscle activation patterns. Although there have been advances in the use of transcutaneous electrical nerve stimulation, it remains extremely challenging to use surface electrodes to provide detailed somatosensory feedback without some pain or discomfort.

In contrast, implanted electrodes have the potential to be highly selective. They may be placed directly inside the nerve where they can record motor commands and stimulate somatosensory feedback with a very high level of precision. Peripheral nerve interfaces are not associated with the same levels of risk as implanted brain interfaces, and neural coding is better understood at the periphery than in the brain or in complex EMG signals [1]. The proximity of the electrodes to the nerve reduces the intensity of stimulation required for axonal excitation, and selective stimulation is possible if using multiple electrode contacts [2]. However, implanting these electrodes requires delicate surgical procedures and there is a real and significant risk of long-term damage to the nerve.

Despite the potential risks, a recent survey of 104 amputees identified that 68% were interested in trying direct peripheral nerve interfaces versus 83% for conventional myoelectric control and 39% for cortical interfaces. Surveyed amputees expressed common concerns about surgical risk and prioritised effective but basic prosthesis features such as opening and closing the hand slowly over more complex features [3].

6.1   Structure of the peripheral nerves

6.1.1   The nervous system

Previous chapters have introduced some of the leading technologies that can be implanted in order to interface with the peripheral nerves. This section will provide a brief overview of the structure and function of the nervous system, with a focus on the neural innervation of the upper limbs.

The brain and spinal cord form the central nervous system (CNS). Extending from these are 12 cranial nerves and 31 spinal nerves that further subdivide to form the PNS. The PNS consists of neurons connecting peripheral receptor and effector organs to each other through the intermediation of the brain and spinal cord.

The PNS contains both the *somatic* and the *autonomic* nervous systems. The somatic nervous system is responsible for voluntary body movements via the skeletal muscles; it includes the nerves responsible for muscle contraction as well as the motor neurons near the skin. Thus, it is of primary interest in nerve interfaces for prosthetic limbs. The autonomic nervous system is responsible for the involuntary bodily functions such as respiration, cardiac function and mucus production. The autonomic nervous system can be further divided into the *sympathetic* and the *parasympathetic* systems [4]. The sympathetic nervous system prepares the body for the fight or flight response, while the parasympathetic nervous system inhibits the body from overworking and restores the body to a calm and composed state.

6.1.2 The nerves of the upper limb

Individual nerve fibres (axons) can be classified by the direction in which they propagate information; motor neurons are termed *efferent* or 'exiting' from the brain and sensory neurons are termed *afferent* or 'entering' the brain. The majority of nerves contain both afferent and efferent fibres, although there is separation at the spinal level where the anterior roots are primarily efferent, and the posterior roots are primarily afferent.

The PNS consists of neurons whose somata are located in the spinal cord or within spinal ganglia; their axons then extend through the peripheral nerves to reach the target organs or muscles. The axons can be either unmyelinated or myelinated, the latter ranging from 2 to 20 μm in diameter, and terminate at the periphery either as free endings or in various specialised sensory receptors. The number and type of nerve fibres is highly variable, depending on the nerve and the anatomical location. Most of the somatic peripheral nerves are mixed, providing motor, sensory and autonomic innervation.

In the hand, movement is produced by over 30 muscles located within the hand (intrinsic) and in the forearm (extrinsic). Innervation of the hand and forearm is shared by the ulnar, median and radial nerves. Intrinsic muscles are responsible for fine motor control and are mostly innervated by terminal branches of the median and ulnar nerves. Extrinsic muscles are responsible for gross flexion and extension of the whole hand and are mostly innervated by the median and radial nerves. Sensory innervation of the hand is provided by the same three nerves, each of which innervates separate but overlapping regions (Figure 6.1).

The median nerve innervates the lateral aspect of the palm, the palmar surface and some of the dorsal surface of the thumb, index and middle finger, along with the palmar surface of the lateral aspect of the ring finger. The ulnar nerve innervates the rest of the palmar surface of the hand, as well as the medial aspect of the dorsal surface of the hand. The radial nerve innervates the rest of the dorsal surface of the hand.

Each of these three nerves contains both afferent and efferent fibres. The efferent fibres innervate muscles and thereby control movement, and the afferent fibres relay information from cutaneous mechanoreceptors, proprioceptors, thermoreceptors and nociceptors back to the spinal cord and brain. Within the wrist, each of the three nerves contains between 20,000 and 35,000 individual nerve fibres in total, the majority of which are afferent as most muscles are proximal to the wrist. The fingertips are most highly innervated by tactile afferent fibres, reflecting their importance for object grasping, manipulation and fine motor control [5].

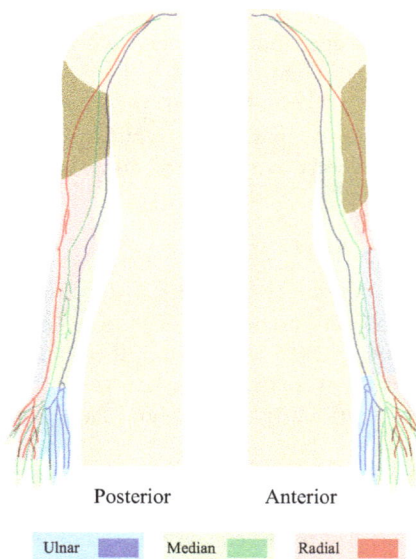

Figure 6.1   *Posterior and anterior sensory innervation of the limbs and hands by the ulnar, median and radial nerves*

6.1.3   *Residual function in peripheral nerve stumps*

The PNS is both mechanically and chemically fragile. Even if a bidirectional nerve interface could be constructed, it would still require an intact and functional proximal nerve. After peripheral nerve injury, there may be changes in the proximal nerve stump, loss of central connections or dynamic changes in cortical areas as a result of CNS plasticity. Among the pathophysiologic changes in the proximal nerve stump, there is greater atrophy of myelinated sensory nerve fibres than of alpha-motor neuron fibres [6]. Tactile and proprioceptive sensations are mediated by large diameter myelinated fibres, and pain sensations are conducted by small diameter myelinated and unmyelinated fibres. Thus, painless tactile sensations can be elicited through focal electrical stimulation of normal intact peripheral nerves because the larger diameter fibres have lower stimulation thresholds than the smaller diameter fibres.

After long-term amputation, the nerve fibres will atrophy and estimates of fibre survivability have varied from 6% to 83%, with a loss of over 50% of alpha-motor neuron cell bodies reported in human amputees [6]. CNS reorganisation begins almost immediately after nerve transection, while functional changes in the nerve stumps are more pronounced after the first 2 months [6]. Dhillon *et al.* have shown that it is possible to record volition motor nerve activity uniquely associated with missing limb movement in long-term (mean 4 year) amputees. Electrical stimulation through the implanted electrodes elicited discrete, unitary, graded sensations of touch, joint movement and position referring to the missing limb.

There is currently limited data on the residual function of peripheral nerve stumps; however, the available findings indicate that the motor and somatosensory pathways retain significant residual connectivity and function for many years after limb amputation.

6.2   Control of prostheses via nerve implants

The previous sections have considered the gross structure of the nervous system, the innervation of the upper limb and the residual function of severed nerve stumps. This section focuses on the principles and approaches for interfacing to these nerves, in order to provide a closed-loop interface for the control of a prosthetic limb. Depending on the application, interfaces with the peripheral nerves must be capable of recording and/or modulating the electrical signals within the axons. In the case of a closed-loop prosthesis both recording and modulating would be required, although these two capabilities need not be fulfilled by the same electrodes.

6.2.1   Principles of neural recording

Obtaining stable chronic recordings from peripheral nerves remains a significant challenge. The electrical signals recorded by the electrodes must be amplified, filtered and processed in order to extract meaningful information for control of the prosthesis. All of these must be done in a way that is resilient to noise and minimises interference from contaminating sources such as muscle activation. Akin to the relationship between invasiveness and selectivity, there exists a similar trend between invasiveness and recorded signal amplitude. Intraneural electrodes might result in signal amplitudes on the order of 100 μV or greater, whereas with cuff electrodes, this amplitude is close to 1–10 μV [7]. At the same time, contaminating signals from nearby muscle activation could be on the order of 1–10 mV. Intraneural electrodes are more likely to record from a single fascicle, or small groups of fascicles, than extraneural electrodes. Further sources of interference include the mains electrical supply, radio-frequency broadcasts and stray magnetic fields.

Processing the recorded signals

These properties lead to one of two distinct situations for processing the recorded signals:

- If the signal amplitudes are large enough and the electrode is sufficiently selective, then it is possible that individual, distinct action potentials can be recorded. These can then be identified and classified based on morphology or conduction velocity (spike sorting), resulting in familiar spike firing raster plots.
- If the signal amplitudes are small and the electrode is not sufficiently selective, then individual action potentials will not be identifiable in the recording. In this case, it may be possible to extract meaningful information by considering spectral approaches, or by extracting amplitude envelopes using statistical measures.

There may be situations where the characteristics of the recorded signal are between these two extremes, and in this case signal processing methods from both domains may be combined [8]. There may be further situations where signals from two different sources, with differing characteristics, are combined for processing. Petrini *et al.* have described an innovative approach in which microneurographic and EMG recordings are combined in order to record human neural signals during activities of motor control, for example [9].

6.2.1.1 Electrode configuration

The most basic recording configuration is the monopole. In this situation, the potential difference between a single recording electrode (placed near, on or in the nerve) and a reference electrode is measured. This arrangement produces large signal amplitudes but the rejection of common-mode interference is poor. Differential, or bipolar, recording decreases the sensitivity of the interface to external noise sources. In the bipolar configuration, two electrodes are connected directly to the inputs of a differential amplifier, with a third reference electrode placed nearby. The recorded signal amplitude now depends largely on the electrode separation as well as the interelectrode impedance [10,11]. A third approach is the tripole configuration in which three amplifiers are used to produce a single recording, as shown in Figure 6.2. The two first-rank amplifiers record differentially between the outer electrodes, and the centre electrode acts as a reference. A third (second-rank) amplifier sums the output signals from the first-rank amplifiers. This arrangement produces the lowest signal amplitudes but has the best resilience to common-mode interference.

The transfer function for a tripole recording arrangement using a cuff electrode provides useful insight into the amplitudes of the recorded signals. This transfer function is given by

$$V_{tp}(t, Z_1, Z_2, Z_3) = \left(\frac{\rho_\epsilon}{\rho_\alpha}\right)\left(\frac{r_a}{r_e}\right)^2\left[V_m\left(t - \frac{Z_1}{v}\right) - 2V_m\left(t - \frac{Z_2}{v}\right) + V_m\left(t - \frac{Z_3}{v}\right)\right],$$

$$(6.1)$$

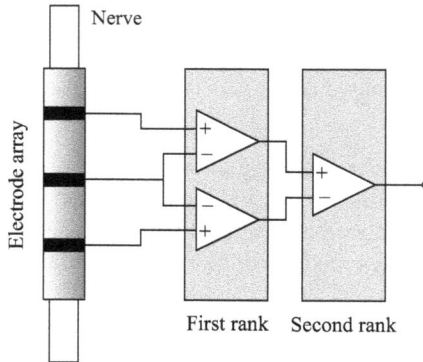

Figure 6.2   The tripolar amplifier configuration illustrated for a three-electrode interface

where $V_m(t)$ is the transmembrane action potential as a function of time, v is the conduction velocity of the action potential, Z_n is the position of each electrode, r_a and r_e are the radii of the axon and the electrode, and ρ_ϵ and ρ_α are the resistivities of the tissue inside the cuff and the axoplasm, respectively [12]. The key observation from this result is that the magnitude of the transfer function is larger for axons with large diameters (and thus faster conduction velocities). In practice, this means that recording from large fibres (such as Aα-motor fibres) is easier than recording from small fibres (such as C fibre nociceptors). The transfer function is also sensitive to the resistivity, and thus impedance, between each electrode. This impedance is time varying in chronically implanted electrodes as encapsulation tissue will eventually form near or around the electrodes. Mismatches in the impedance between different electrodes will also degrade the common-mode signal rejection performance.

6.2.1.2 Amplification

Amplification is a crucial component of any recording system, the goal being to increase the signal amplitudes from a handful of micro-volts to a few volts without adding any noise in the process. This amplification is required in order to ensure sufficient signal-to-noise ratios (SNRs) later in the processing chain (e.g. before analogue-to-digital conversion). In practice, even the best low-noise amplifiers will contribute some noise to the recording. For example, at the time of writing, the best commercial instrumentation amplifiers have voltage noise densities of around 1 nV/$\sqrt{Hz}^{1/2}$ and current noise densities of around 1.5 pA/$\sqrt{Hz}^{1/2}$, considering typical neural signal bandwidth (10 Hz–10 kHz) and electrode impedance (1 kΩ), this easily leads to noise floors of a few micro-volts.*

6.2.2 Signal processing methods

Once the electrical activity within the nerve has been recorded, it must be filtered and processed. Filtering can serve two purposes; to remove interference artefacts and to remove instrumentation noise. The filtering approach must be designed for the specific system, but, broadly speaking, the typical approaches include (a) analogue bandpass filters that are integrated within the amplification and recording electronics, (b) adaptive mains rejection filters, (c) discrete time digital filters and (d) wavelet denoising.

6.2.2.1 Temporal methods

Processing of the recorded neural signals is dependant on the geometry and number of the electrodes, as well as the SNR. The most basic method is to compute the average amplitude or power within the signal; this can be done by computing the RMS or the variance of the signal using a sliding time window. The length of the window and the overlap from one window to another should be chosen based on the expected rate of change of the signal. For example, Jezernik *et al.* utilised both a simple low-pass

---

*Analog Devices AD8429 Datasheet.

filter and a sliding RMS window to extract information about bladder fullness from the extradural sacral roots [13].

If the SNR is high enough, and the interface selective enough, then individual action potentials (in this context called *spikes*) can be detected and classified based on morphology. This method borrows techniques from CNS recordings and is commonly called 'spike-sorting'. The basic procedure in spike sorting is (a) detect each spike in the recording using a threshold, (b) extract data windows, each of which should contain a single spike and should be aligned based on a feature such as the spike's peak or centroid, (c) reduce the number of samples required for classification using, for example, principal component analysis and (d) classify each spike using conventional clustering approaches [14]. The output of the spike-sorting process is a raster plot of spike events that can then be used to extract information (see Figure 6.5 for an example of this process).

Another method is velocity discrimination, which is based on the fact that the conduction velocity of the action potential is a function of the axon properties and can be used to classify action potentials as they propagate. Recordings must be made by electrodes that are spaced equidistantly along the length of the nerve. The essence of velocity discrimination is a simple process called delay-and-add, that is analogous to the beam-forming algorithms used in certain types of synthetic aperture arrays [15]. The signals recorded from each electrode are delayed relative to one another by an interval that corresponds to the conduction velocity of interest and then summed together [16].

One advantage of this process is the ability to record separately neural activity that is both afferent and efferent by simply applying a negative value of delay. Furthermore, when delay-and-add is used and the noise sources are uncorrelated, there is an increase in SNR of approximately $\sqrt{N}$, where N is the number of electrodes [17]. This property can be exploited to identify action potentials that may not be observable directly in the time records of the individual channels and thus could not be classified by traditional methods such as spike-sorting. Velocity discrimination has been used successfully to record naturally occurring afferent signals in the vagus nerve of pig and the dorsal roots of rat [18,19]. In the dorsal roots of rat, a six-electrode array was attached to the L5 dorsal root, and velocity discrimination was used to observe changes in the firing rates of individual fibres in response to manual cutaneous stimulation. An example of the raster plot output provided by this method is shown in Figure 6.3; in this illustration, the shaded box indicates cutaneous stimulation.

6.2.2.2   Spatial methods

There are other signal processing methods that can extract spatial information from peripheral nerve recordings using electrodes placed around the nerve. The first of these is based on flat-interface nerve electrode (FINE)-type cuffs and extends methods for antenna array beamforming. Linear, time-invariant, real-valued weights are applied to the voltage recorded at each contact on the FINE nerve cuff electrode to shape the receptive field within the nerve. The algorithm is based on a priori knowledge of the cuff geometry. This approach produces a heat map that localises activity to individual

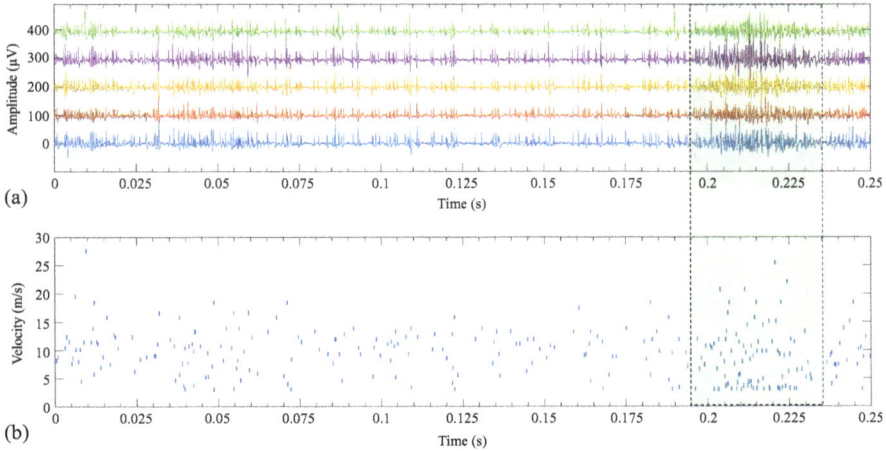

Figure 6.3 *(a) Time domain recordings from a six-electrode array fitted to the L5 dorsal root of a rat, (b) action potentials detected using velocity discrimination of the recordings; the shaded box indicates cutaneous stimulation*

fascicles and has been applied to fascicle selective recording from the sciatic nerve of dog using a 16-electrode FINE with promising results [20,21].

Another method that provides fascicular-level selectivity using electrodes distributed around the nerve is electrical impedance tomography (EIT). In this method, a flexible, cylindrical, multi-electrode cuff is placed around a nerve, and the medical imaging technique of fast EIT is applied to image the activity within the fascicles. A pilot study has been carried out in the sciatic nerve of rat and has shown that it is possible to distinguish separate fascicles activated in response to direct electrical stimulation of the posterior tibial and common peroneal nerves; an illustration of this process is shown in Figure 6.4. This approach is significantly more selective than inverse source analysis but as yet has only been demonstrated on electrically evoked compound action potentials rather than naturally occurring neural signals [22].

Despite the significant promise offered by the more advanced temporally and spatially selective signal processing methods, none have yet been applied to extracting volitional motor activity from peripheral nerves for the control of prostheses. Only amplitude/power and conventional spike sorting have been applied for this purpose, and these examples will now be discussed in more detail.

6.2.3 Direct ENG-based control

Information extracted from the efferent pathways of the median, ulnar and radial nerves can be translated into movement commands and used to drive a prosthesis directly. Both implanted and percutaneous electrodes have been used for this purpose

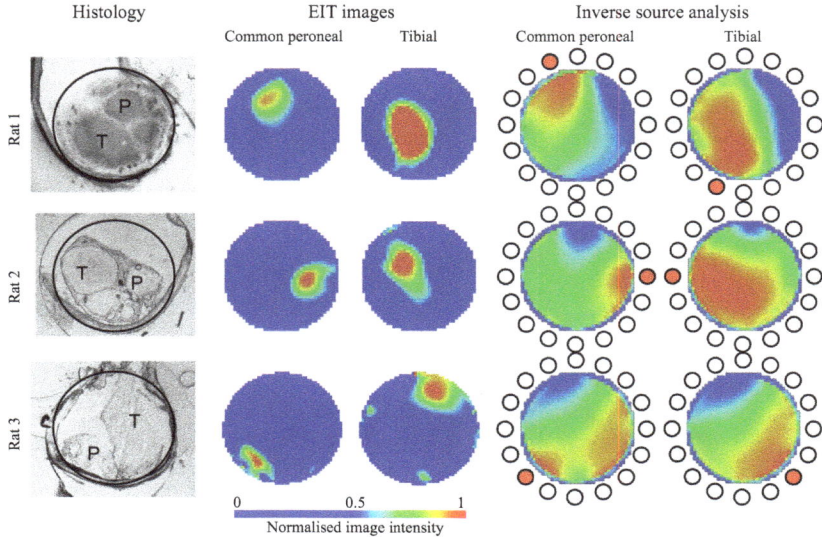

Figure 6.4   EIT images of the sciatic nerve overlap with morphological localisation of tibial (T) and peroneal (P) fascicles in rat. Reproduced from [22]

and more recently have been combined with simultaneous EMG recordings to perform hybrid processing.

Some of the earliest work to demonstrate volitional motor control by direct neural interfacing was performed by Dhillon *et al.* [6] by means of longitudinally implanted intrafascicular electrodes (LIFEs) implanted within a healthy portion of the median and/or the ulnar nerve proximal to any terminal neuroma. Recordings were made in a bipolar configuration and amplified ($G = 20,000$), bandpass-filtered (0.3 Hz–4 kHz) and connected to both a loudspeaker and a recording device. The subjects were directed to produce the loudest audible change in sound by performing imagined arm movement of the severed limb. Findings indicated that it was possible to record volitional motor nerve activity uniquely associated with missing limb movements based on the amplitude envelope of the recorded signals.

More recently, Rossini *et al.* demonstrated a bidirectional peripheral nerve interface in which motor activity was recorded from a 26-year-old male subject with severely atrophied stump muscles that were non-functional for EMG control [23]. Two thin-film LIFEs (tf-LIFE4s) were implanted into both the ulnar and medial nerves following epineural micro-dissection [24]. The experimental protocol included four phases that encompassed the recording of the motor output in order to control the hand and sensory stimulation of afferent fibres to elicit sensation.

Neural signals electroneurogram (ENG) were recorded with ($G = 10,000$) and bandpass-filtered (100 Hz–10 kHz). Online processing of the ENG was performed by computing mean rectified values over data windows of 1,000 samples with a sample rate of 48 kHz. In the later phases of the study, the ENG channels within the tf-LIFE4s that gave the best SNRs were selected for offline analysis in order to improve the sensitivity and specificity of the signal processing. Two main approaches were used: (a) selected features from the ENG were extracted and fed into an artificial neural network for the identification of motor command onset, and (b) wavelet denoising of the measured ENG and conventional spike-sorting using a template creation and matching approach. Finally, a support vector machine was used to infer the type of movement based on the wave forms of the identified spikes. The implemented method for interpreting the motor commands and controlling the prosthesis is shown in Figure 6.5.

The SNR of the implanted tf-LIFE increased during the post-surgery period, stabilising after 10 days. The tf-LIFE4s were implanted for 4 weeks and remained stable over that time period. Simultaneous recording from multiple electrode sites in both median and ulnar nerve improved the rate of correct classification for movement control with higher sensitivity and specificity when compared to single electrode site recording. The correct classification of each movement was improved with learning from 75% to 85% over a 2-day period.

Clark *et al.* implanted two 100-electrode Utah Slanted Electrode Arrays (USEAs) in the median and ulnar nerves of an amputee for 4 weeks [25]. During the experiment, the impedances of functioning electrodes remained stable, although interference from muscle activity often occluded the ENG. It was possible to use the USEAs to control one to two degrees of freedom.

Petrini *et al.* have described a new hybrid method to record and characterise motor efferents recorded using microneurography during voluntary isokinetic and isotonic hand movements. The authors simultaneously recorded neural signals from the median nerve and surface Electromyography (sEMG) signals from multiple muscles in the lower arm. They successfully recorded a variety of signals that were related to different force levels, velocities of movement execution and different types of grasping. They also showed, in simulation, that the extracted signal features would be consistent if recorded from an implantable transverse intrafascicular multichannel electrode (TIME) intraneural electrode in amputees [9].

The limited number of studies that explore directly the use of implantable nerve interfaces for the control of prostheses in humans is almost certainly linked to the difficulties in obtaining stable and good-quality recordings. The PNS is a relatively hostile environment compared to the CNS; movement in the recording area causes issues with interference, damage to electrodes, and changes in signal amplitudes (via changes in distance from electrode to axon). There have been significantly more studies that demonstrate sensory feedback through neural stimulation, as will be discussed later in this chapter.

6.2.4 Targeted muscle reinnervation

A different approach to the direct neural control of prostheses is targeted muscle reinnervation (TMR). TMR increases the amount of information that can be extracted from the peripheral nerves by surgically attaching the proximal nerve stump to residual muscles. The efferent pathways in the nerve stump then form functional connections

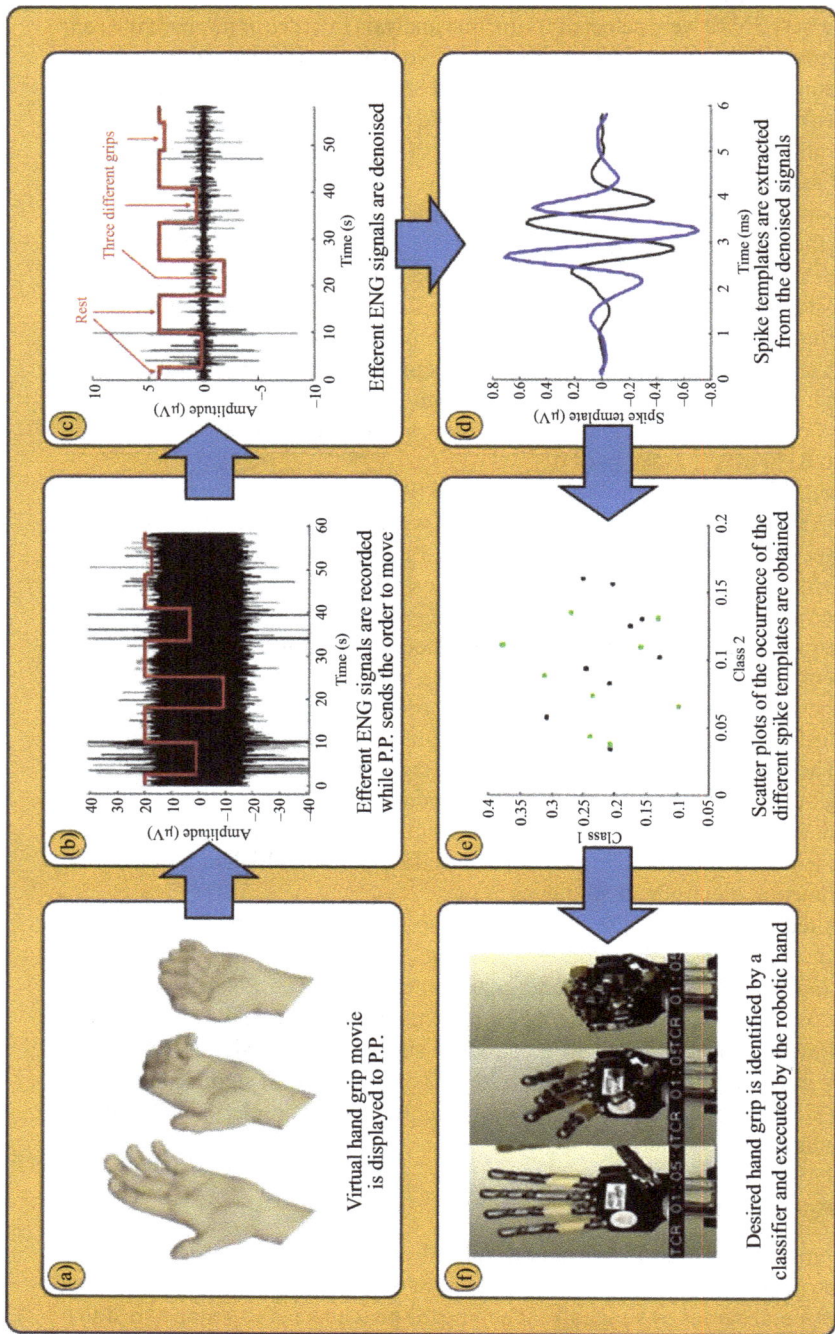

Figure 6.5   Example processing scheme for recording, identifying and classifying volitional motor activity from tf-LIFE4s implanted in the median and ulnar nerves. (a) virtual hand grasping; (b) recording and pre-processing; (c) de-noising; (d) feature extraction; (e) selection of the motor command; (f) control of the prosthesis. Reproduced from [23].

(reinnervate) to the residual muscles in 3–6 months. In this way, the small, difficult to detect motor signals in the peripheral nerve may instead be detected by EMG electrodes placed over the reinnervated muscles. Apart from the initial surgery to attach the proximal stump to the residual muscles, the process is non-invasive as surface electrodes are used to record the EMG. If sufficient residual muscle is available, multiple EMG recording sites can be used to obtain multiple simultaneous control functions, such as hand opening and closing and elbow flexion and tension. TMR is a clinically available procedure and has been performed on more than 40 upper limb amputees worldwide [26].

6.3   Sensory restoration via nerve implants

Having considered the various approaches to recording volitional motor commands from peripheral nerves, this section will focus on the principles and methods for stimulating nerves in order to provide somatosensory feedback from a prosthetic limb.

6.3.1   Principles of electrical stimulation

Electrical stimulation has been applied to the PNS for many decades, and there are now a multitude of implantable clinical devices that operate on this principle. These include a vagus nerve simulator for the treatment of drug restive epilepsy, the Brindley sacral anterior root stimulation system, a neuromodulation technique used for management of the urinary bladder first introduced in 1972 [27] and the cardiac pacemaker.

When electrical currents are delivered to the peripheral nerves, there are two possible outcomes: (a) the current creates a potential field that can alter the state of the voltage-gated ion channels and trigger the generation of action potentials, and (b) the current causes uncontrolled electrochemical reactions that can cause damage to the electrode or injury to the nerve [28]. The principles of electrical stimulation must guide the design of devices that can selectively generate action potentials without causing long-lasting damage. It is also possible to use electrical stimulation to *block* the conduction of action potentials, although further discussion of this effect is beyond the scope of this chapter.

Electrical stimulation is achieved by connecting a stimulus source to the tissue via electrodes. The number of electrodes can vary but there must be at least two, the *anode* and the *cathode*, between which current may flow. The characteristics of the stimulus applied to the nerve can be measured by its voltage or its current, and these are both time-varying. The current or voltage will most likely take the form of a pulse, with an associated amplitude, duration and shape (triangular, sinusoidal or rectangular). The surface area of the electrode tissue interface will determine the charge and current density, which decrease with increasing surface area and distance from the electrode to the axon. The threshold required for an axon to generate an action potential is inversely proportional to diameter, i.e. large axons have a lower stimulation threshold.

During stimulation, charge transfer can be either potentiostatic (voltage controlled) or galvanostatic (current controlled). The latter is preferred as it enables direct control of the charge injected, and the membrane potential depends directly on the applied current rather than the applied voltage [29]. It is also more convenient to consider the stimulus in terms of the charge density, as this is more readily linked to known stimulation thresholds.

6.3.2   Stimulation waveforms and safety

There are advantages and disadvantages of using stimulation waveforms that feature non-square pulses. The waveform has an important role in the efficiency, selectivity and safety of electrical stimulation. Stimulation efficiency is very important for conserving battery power in implanted devices, and the complex relationship between energy, charge and power efficiency has led to the development of complex pulse shapes. An optimal energy-efficient waveform was found using a genetic algorithm and approaches a truncated Gaussian shape [30].

In terms of selectivity, there is significant interest in identifying stimulation waveforms that enable the selective stimulation of specific fibre types, essentially overcoming the inverse recruitment characteristics of the axon. Quasitrapezoidal pulses have been shown to be selective when stimulating the vagus nerve and in the control of the urinary bladder and exponential rising waveforms have shown increased size selectivity in motor fibres [31].

In terms of safety, with constant current stimulation, it is preferable to use *bi-phasic* waveforms. Bi-phasic stimuli have both positive and corresponding negative phases of charge transfer in order to recover reversible injected charge and avoid drift in the potential; the area under the curve of each phase represents the total charge injected. It is not always possible to recover all of the injected charge and so the two phases may not be exactly balanced. The applied stimulus must not cause damage to either the stimulating electrodes or the target tissue, and although the exact mechanisms that underlie stimulation-induced injury of peripheral nerve remain unclear, there have been attempts to define safe operating regions. Shannon *et al.* introduced a model based on empirical data that defines a line separating stimulation regimes that are known to cause damage from those that are not. This line is given by

$$\log\left(\frac{Q}{A}\right) = k - \log(Q) \tag{6.2}$$

where Q/A is the charge density (the charge per phase over the geometric surface area of the electrode) and k is an empirically defined constant [32]. This is a useful model for situations similar to those in which the empirical data were collected, but there are other factors that have the potential for tissue damage, such as repetition frequency, current density, electrode size and materials and variations in the target tissue (CNS versus PNS) [33].

6.3.3 Direct neural stimulation

As far back as the 1970s, there have been attempts to produce sensations via cuff or needle electrodes by applying electrical stimulation directly to the nerves [34]. In these early attempts, the subjects typically reported paraesthesia, vibration or pulsing spread across the phantom hand. Of course the ideal sensory feedback mechanism would provide the same perception as the original limb. Recent work has shown that by optimising both the electrode and the stimulation waveform, it is possible to produce sensations of touch, pressure and movement at more precise locations.

The basic paradigm for sensory restoration is to implant an electrode into or onto the residual nerve, apply different stimulation waveforms and then ask the subject for verbal reports or psychophysical judgements of sensation. Modulation of the stimulation waveforms can include changes in amplitude (intensity), pulse duration, stimulation frequency and waveform shape. The large number of parameters represents one of the main challenges associated with electrical stimulation, and many studies have explored the parameter space to understand how to map feedback to specific sensations.

Stimulation may also be applied through different electrodes in order to selectively stimulate different fascicles and thus modulate the perception. Stimulation through different electrodes can also evoke sensations with different qualities, dependent on the type of receptor that the fibres formally innervated [1,35]. It might be expected that intrafascicular electrodes would provide greater spatial localisation of the perceived sensations, but in fact both intra- and extrafascicular stimulations have shown similar receptive fields [36].

Recent studies of sensory restoration using implanted neural stimulation have attempted both unidirectional (sensory only) or bidirectional control of prosthetic hands. Raspopovic *et al.* implanted four TIMEs in the median and ulnar nerves (two electrodes in each) of a single amputee [36]. The aim was to restore the sense of touch in a transradial amputee by means of electrical stimulation via the TIMEs. This bidirectional interface relied on myoelectric sensing of the efferent pathways and a feedback loop for stimulating the afferent pathways directly. Initially, the medial and ulnar nerves were stimulated with different patterns in order to identify all of the possible sensations and their referred locations. The myographic control pathway was then enabled, allowing the amputee to both move the prosthesis and feel feedback from sensors embedded within the prosthesis.

The tactile sensory feedback was evaluated over a 4-week period to measure the stability of the elicited sensations. The stimulus was a train of cathodic rectangular biphasic pulses, the train had a pulse repetition frequency of 50 Hz and a duration of 500 ms. The injected charge was varied over the duration, with thresholds from slight contact to mild pain ranging from 14 to 24 nC for the median nerve and 4 to 8 nC for the ulnar nerve. The amputee was able to control three different levels of exerted pressure with the index and little finger with a success rate > 90%. Importantly, the performance of the prosthetic hand was compared to the healthy hand and demonstrated that direct sensory feedback was more effective than just visual and auditory feedback for the same task.

A long-term experimental study has been performed by Tan *et al.* in which two amputees were involved in order to demonstrate the elicitation of tactile sensory feedback for up to 24 months [37]. The effect of this sensory feedback on task performance was assessed in the later work by Schiefer *et al.* [38]. The two amputees were implanted with different electrode configurations: (1) two 8-contact FINE electrodes, one each in the median and ulnar nerves, and one spiral electrode in the radial, and (2) two 8-contact FINE electrodes, one each in the median and radial nerves. Force and bend sensors were fitted to the thumb, index and middle finger of an Ottobock Sensor-Hand Speed to generate sensor data, and the hand was controlled using myoelectric signals.

Different stimulation strategies were employed using time-invariant parameters and time-variant pulse widths. The use of patterned stimulation intensities, hypothesised to introduce information into the peripheral nerves by population coding, controlled the quality of sensory perception. The elicited sensations were described by the amputees and the involved areas are shown in Figure 6.6; these areas show general agreement with the known anatomical innervation of the median, ulnar and radial nerves. In both subjects, the elicited sensations and the referred locations on the phantom limb were stable and repeatable throughout the study.

Ortiz-Catalan *et al.* performed another long-term experimental study in which tactile sensory feedback was elicited for 11 months in a single subject using a three-channel cuff electrode implanted on the ulnar nerve [39]. The prosthetic hand was controlled by myoelectric signals recorded using epimysial electrodes. Tactile sensory feedback was elicited in three distinct areas on the phantom limb and was stable over the 11 months of the experiment. Biphasic and charge-balanced pulses were used as a stimulation waveform, superficial tapping was felt for frequencies

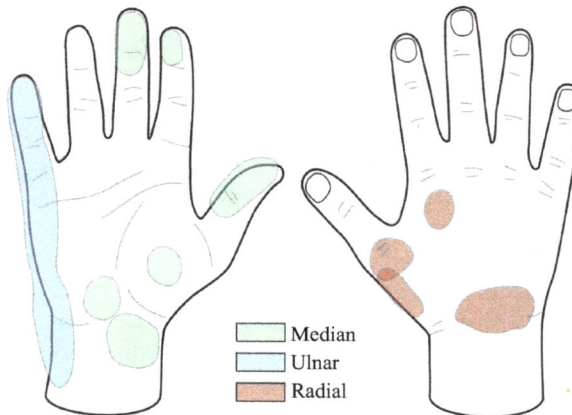

Figure 6.6   Exemplar sensation locations achievable using FINE or cuff electrodes implanted on either the Median, Ulnar, or Radial Nerves. Based on results obtained 3 weeks post-operation from [37]

between 8 and 10 Hz, and tingling above 20 Hz. Increasing the stimulation current from 30 to 50 μA increased the size of the receptive area as did increasing the frequency. The sensory feedback had the effect of improving both the controllability of the prosthesis and the duration of usage, it also reduced phantom limb pain by 40%.

6.3.4   Interfaces with the dorsal root ganglia

Instead of stimulating the residual peripheral nerve in the upper limb, it is possible to implant electrodes in the dorsal root ganglia (DRG), located close to the spinal cord within the intervertebral foramina [40]. Surgery to access the DRG is more complicated than accessing the peripheral nerves in the arm and requires a laminectomy. However, this surgery is very similar to that routinely performed in order to implant the sacral anterior root stimulator for urinary bladder control [41]. One complication of stimulating the DRG is that although the sensory innervation of the hand is served by three dorsal roots, these roots do not intuitively map onto the median, ulnar and radial nerves. Thus, full sensory innervation would still require at least three electrodes to be implanted in three locations. Sensory feedback could then be achieved by identifying the optimal stimulation patterns for each root. However, a key advantage is that the DRG only contains afferent fibres and so it is less likely that stimulation will inadvertently recruit efferent fibres.

6.3.5   Biomimetic feedback

Despite the significant promise shown with direct neural stimulation, it has been difficult to systematically elicit sensations that are stable and of specific quality. The biomimetic approach relies on a deeper understanding of how mechanical forces applied to the skin are ordinarily translated into afferent signals and by modelling this translation can provide a more natural sensations. The mechanoreceptors in the human skin facilitate sensing forces, patterns and slip. The compliance of the skin enables it to indent and stretch in response to external pressure and contour, stimulating the mechanoreceptors at and around the contact region.

There are four types of mechanoreceptors in the skin of the hand, and these fall into four classes based on their adaptation speed and depth in the skin. Markel cells (SA1) and Ruffini endings (SA2) are slow adapting and they respond to applied pressure and skin stretch, respectively. Meissner corpuscle (RA1) and Pacinian corpuscle (RA1) are fast adapting, and they are stimulated by lateral motion and vibrations, respectively. Figure 6.7 illustrates this relationship.

Each of the four mechanoreceptors plays an important role during the grasping of an object. SA1 measures the applied force throughout the grasp duration to ensure that the right force is applied. SA2 detects the skin sketch, allowing monitoring of the finger extension and flexion. RA1 and RA2 are stimulated at the beginning and the end of the grasp, sensing the speed of the grasp and when the object leaves and touches the surface, respectively.

When the hand is in contact with an object, the four types of afferents are activated to convey information about the object's texture, shape, size and motion.

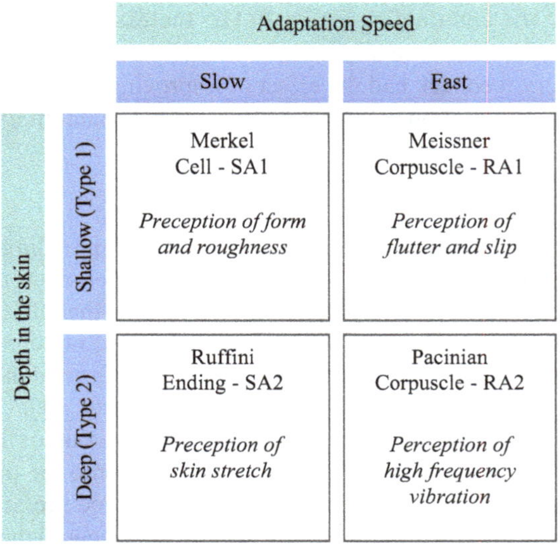

Adaptation Speed		
	Slow	**Fast**
Shallow (Type 1)	Merkel Cell - SA1 *Preception of form and roughness*	Meissner Corpuscle - RA1 *Perception of flutter and slip*
Deep (Type 2)	Ruffini Ending - SA2 *Preception of skin stretch*	Pacinian Corpuscle - RA2 *Perception of high frequency vibration*

Figure 6.7   Skin deformation is sensed by four types of mechanoreceptors in the skin: Markel cells (SA1) and Ruffini endings (SA2) are slow adapting, while Meissner Corpuscle (RA1) and Pacinian Corpuscle (RA1 or PC) are fast adapting

Saal *et al.* have developed tools that model peripheral nerve coding and attempt to produce stimulation waveforms that more accurately elicit neural coding typical of genuine sensation. As an example of this, they have examined the effect of skin indentation by modelling the spiking dynamics generated by the innervating SA1, RA and PC fibres. Although this study did not consider the SA2 fibres, and contains a number of other simplifications, this model can be employed to define peripheral stimulation patterns for tactile stimuli. An example of this model is shown in Figure 6.8, in which a simple dynamic skin indentation is shown to produce different neural responses from the SA1, RA and PC receptors (according to their function); these responses are then combined to form a more realistic population response for all fibres.

The ability to recreate the neural coding is dependant on the availability of a sufficient number of sensors on the prosthesis, and on the stability and selectivity of the implanted electrodes. The computational complexity of the model must also be considered, although simplified models have been proposed [43].

TouchSim, developed by Saal *et al.*, is a detailed model that receives an input of the static and dynamic pressure applied at each sensor position, uses this to set the 13 different parameters of leaky integrate-and-fire models, as shown in Figure 6.9, and produces a spiking pattern for each of the afferents in the population [44].

Biomimetic encoding has been tested on human subjects using a multitude of different electrodes and sensors. Valle *et al.* assessed the naturalness and discriminability

Dynamic skin indentation   Neural response   Biomimetic
population response

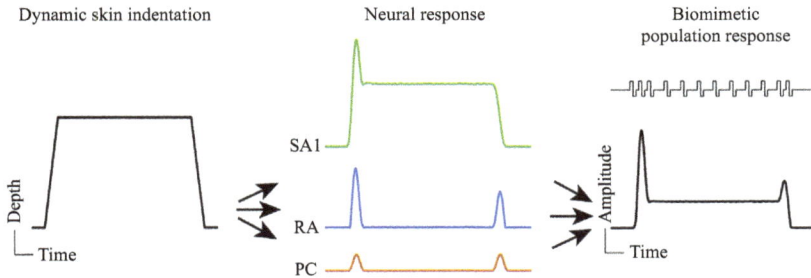

Figure 6.8   Conveying dynamic pressure signals through biomimetic peripheral nerve stimulation. Reproduced from [1]

of sensations elicited by TIMEs in two transradial amputees using four encoding methods, as well as the reported embodiment and improved functional performance. The different encoding methods that are shown included linear amplitude neuromodulation (ANM), frequency neuromodulation (FNM) and two hybrid neuromodulation (HNM-1, HNM-2) paradigms. FNM uses TouchSim to modulate the frequency to create a biomimetic pulse. Both hybrid mechanisms include both frequency and amplitude modulation. The first combines ANM and FNM, while the second modulates the magnitude based on the recruitment of fibres predicted by TouchSim. The results of the experiment showed that hybrid solutions, relying on both frequency and amplitude modulation, were most effective. This is thought to be due to frequency encoding providing the natural sensation and amplitude modulation increasing the discriminability of the sensations [45].

6.3.6   Targeted sensory reinnervation

Another approach to sensory feedback is targeted sensory reinnervation (TSR) [1]. TSR does not require a direct interface with the peripheral nerve but instead relies on surgically attaching the proximal nerve stump to residual skin. This approach is analogous to TMI except that the nerve stump reinnervates a patch of skin rather than a residual muscle. The afferent pathways in the nerve stump then form functional connections (reinnervate) to the skin [46]. Touching the reinnervated site will then elicit sensations that are experienced at the former termination site of the nerve fibres. However, this sensation is somatotopically innervated and so neighbouring areas of the newly innervated skin will not provide sensations from neighbouring areas of the former limb, although the sensitivity to touch is similar. The reinnervated site can then be stimulated using an array of small actuators to provide sensory feedback from a prosthesis, the limiting factors being the limited spatial resolution of the reinnervated skin area and the actuator array. Apart from the initial surgery to attach the proximal stump to the skin, the process is non-invasive as no electrodes or devices are implanted. The interface is stable in the long term and the perceived sensations feel natural without the tingling or paraesthesia that can occur with direct electrical stimulation.

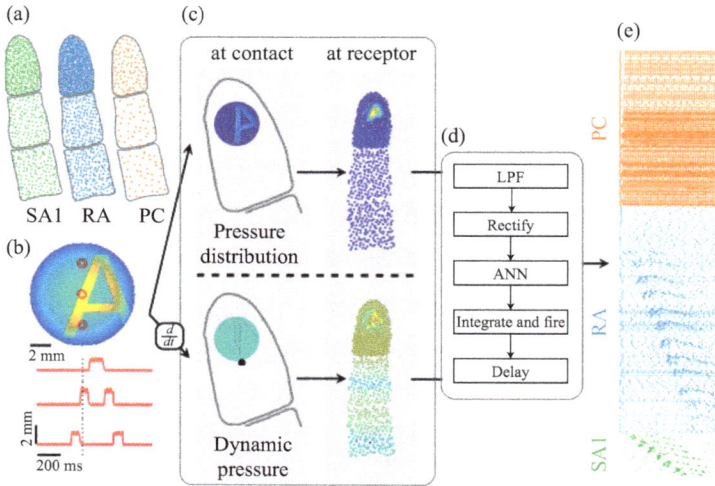

Figure 6.9   Illustration of biomimetic model operation. (a) The density-based distribution of the different afferents. (b) The tactile stimulus applied, resulting in static and dynamic change in pressure as shown in (c). (d) The response of the different afferents is determined by a multi-process model. (e) Output of the model. Modified from [44]

6.4   Summary

This chapter has reviewed the basic principles behind electrical interfaces to the PNS for the purpose of direct neural control of an upper limb prosthetic. Current research efforts in this field have revealed the potential benefits associated with a bidirectional neural interface to the residual peripheral nerves. Such an interface could directly derive volitional motor intention by recording from the efferent fibres and can elicit detailed and time-invariant tactile sensation by stimulating the afferent fibres.

6.4.1   Simultaneous control and sensory restoration

There have been relatively few attempts to produce an interface that simultaneously enables control of a prosthetic and provides sensory restoration at the same time. One of the most successful of these attempts demonstrated restoration of motor control and both proprioceptive and cutaneous sensation in two individuals with upper limb amputation via multiple USEAs [47]. Two 100-electrode USEAs were implanted for 4–5 weeks, one each in the median and ulnar nerves. Intended finger and wrist positions were decoded from neural firing patterns using a modified Kalman filter. Stimulation via the USEAs was additionally used to evoke numerous sensory precepts spanning the phantom hand. In the case of closed-loop control, the ulnar-nerve USEA was used for stimulation, while the median-nerve USEA was used for recording.

This approach was able to provide the subjects with five degrees of freedom of control and up to 131 distinct proprioceptive and cutaneous percepts across the subjects' phantom hands. One subject was provided with limited closed-loop control of a virtual hand – the first demonstration of a closed-loop control of a hand in transradial amputees. In both subjects, the number of working electrodes (as measured by electrode impedance) was variable, and in the case of two USEAs declined rapidly over time, highlighting the difficulty of long-term implantation in the periphery.

6.4.2 Future challenges

Despite the potential advantages of an implanted bidirectional neural interface, there remain several key challenges that include both technological and regulatory issues. Improvements in the design and manufacture of electrodes have enabled short-to-medium-term implantation, although further advances are needed to develop the miniaturised and wireless electrodes to remove the need for percutaneous connectors or wires. There have been many studies that have demonstrated effective and stable restoration of tactile sensory feedback, and advances in this area will likely involve the further development of biomimetic techniques that aim to improve the realism and specificity of the feedback. At the same time, it will be necessary to develop new sensors that can provide highly sensitive and fast observations of applied pressure.

In the majority of the studies reviewed in this chapter, the recording of volitional motor activity was performed using EMG, which is a direct reflection on the ease of use of this method and its relatively good performance. However, the ideal bidirectional interface would also record from the efferent fibres directly. Recording from large populations of fibres, using a chronically implantable interface, remains a significant technological challenge. Relatively, few studies on the neural control of upper limb prostheses have attempted to use direct neural recording, and this is reflective of the difficulty of making stable recordings. There have been a number of key developments in neural recording from other areas in the periphery, such as the introduction of techniques like EIT and velocity discrimination, that could be adapted to the nerves of the upper limb. Such techniques, combined with improvement of electrode stability, could be used to improve the performance of long-term neural recording systems.

References

[1]   Saal HP and Bensmaia SJ. Biomimetic approaches to bionic touch through a peripheral nerve interface. Neuropsychologia. 2015;79:344–353. Available from: http://dx.doi.org/10.1016/j.neuropsychologia.2015.06.010.

[2]   Navarro X, Krueger TB, Lago N, Micera S, Stieglitz T, and Dario P. A critical review of interfaces with the peripheral nervous system for the control of neuroprostheses and hybrid bionic systems. Journal of the Peripheral Nervous System: JPNS. 2005;10(3):229–258. Available from: http://www.ncbi.nlm.nih.gov/pubmed/16221284.

[3]   Engdahl SM, Christie BP, Kelly B, Davis A, Chestek CA, and Gates DH. Surveying the interest of individuals with upper limb loss in novel prosthetic control techniques. Journal of NeuroEngineering and Rehabilitation. 2015;12(1):1–11. Available from: http://dx.doi.org/10.1186/s12984-015-0044-2.

[4]   Williams P, Warick R, Dyson M, and Bannister L. Major divisions of the nervous system. In: Gray's Anatomy. 37th ed.; London: Churchill Livingstone, Inc., 1989. p. 919.

[5]   Vallbo AB and Johansson RS. Properties of cutaneous mechanoreceptors in the human hand related to touch sensation. Human Neurobiology. 1984;3(1):3–14.

[6]   Dhillon GS, Lawrence SM, Hutchinson DT, and Horch KW. Residual function in peripheral nerve stumps of amputees: implications for neural control of artificial limbs. Journal of Hand Surgery. 2004;29(4):605–615.

[7]   Metcalfe BW, Nielsen TN, Donaldson NdN, Hunter AJ, and Taylor JT. First demonstration of velocity selective recording from the pig vagus using a nerve cuff shows respiration afferents. Biomedical Engineering Letters. 2018;8(1):127–136. Available from: http://link.springer.com/10.1007/s13534-017-0054-z.

[8]   Raspopovic S, Cimolato A, Panarese A, *et al.* Neural signal recording and processing in somatic neuroprosthetic applications. A review. Journal of Neuroscience Methods. 2020;337:108653. Available from: https://linkinghub.elsevier.com/retrieve/pii/S0165027020300753.

[9]   Petrini FM, Mazzoni A, Rigosa J, *et al.* Microneurography as a tool to develop decoding algorithms for peripheral neuro-controlled hand prostheses. BioMedical Engineering OnLine. 2019;18(1):1–22. Available from: https://doi.org/10.1186/s12938-019-0659-9.

[10]   Donaldson N, Taylor J, and Winter J. Velocity-selective recording using multi-electrode nerve cuffs. In: Proc 7th IFESS Conference; 2002. p. 1–3. Available from: http://ifess.org/proceedings/IFESS2002/IFESS2002_041_Donaldson.pdf.

[11]   Brunton E, Blau C, and Nazarpour K. Separability of neural responses to standardised mechanical stimulation of limbs. Scientific Reports. 2017;7:11138.

[12]   Taylor J, Donaldson N, and Winter J. Multiple-electrode nerve cuffs for low-velocity and velocity-selective neural recording. Medical & Biological Engineering & Computing. 2004;42(5):634–643. Available from: http://link.springer.com/10.1007/BF02347545.

[13]   Jezernik S, Wen J, and Rijkhoff N. Whole nerve cuff recordings from nerves innervating the urinary bladder. In: Second Annual IFESS; 1997. Available from: http://ifess.org/proceedings/IFESS1997/IFESS1997_024_Jezernik.pdf.

[14]   Gibson S, Judy JW, and Markovic D. Spike sorting: the first step in decoding the brain: the first step in decoding the brain. IEEE Signal Processing Magazine. 2012;29(1):124–143. Available from: http://ieeexplore.ieee.org/lpdocs/epic03/wrapper.htm?arnumber=6105476.

[15] Huang Y and Miller JP. Phased-array processing for spike discrimination. Journal of Neurophysiology. 2004;92(3):1944–1957. Available from: http://www.ncbi.nlm.nih.gov/pubmed/15115796.

[16] Taylor J, Schuettler M, Clarke C, and Donaldson N. The theory of velocity selective neural recording: a study based on simulation. Medical & Biological Engineering & Computing. 2012;50(3):309–318. Available from: http://www.ncbi.nlm.nih.gov/pubmed/22362024.

[17] Donaldson N, Rieger R, Schuettler M, and Taylor J. Noise and selectivity of velocity-selective multi-electrode nerve cuffs. Medical & Biological Engineering & Computing. 2008;46(10):1005–1018. Available from: http://www.ncbi.nlm.nih.gov/pubmed/18696136.

[18] Metcalfe B, Nielsen T, and Taylor J. Velocity selective recording: a demonstration of effectiveness on the vagus nerve in pig. In: 2018 40th Annual International Conference of the IEEE Engineering in Medicine and Biology Society (EMBC). IEEE; 2018. p. 1–4. Available from: https://ieeexplore.ieee.org/document/8512991/.

[19] Metcalfe BW, Chew DJ, Clarke CT, Donaldson NdN, and Taylor JT. A new method for spike extraction using velocity selective recording demonstrated with physiological ENG in rat. Journal of Neuroscience Methods. 2015;251:47–55. Available from: http://www.ncbi.nlm.nih.gov/pubmed/25983203.

[20] Dweiri YM, Eggers TE, Gonzalez-Reyes LE, Drain J, McCallum GA, and Durand DM. Stable detection of movement intent from peripheral nerves: chronic study in dogs. Proceedings of the IEEE. 2017;105(1):50–65.

[21] Wodlinger B and Durand DM. Localization and recovery of peripheral neural sources with beamforming algorithms. IEEE Transactions on Neural Systems and Rehabilitation Engineering. 2009;17(5):461–468. Available from: https://linkinghub.elsevier.com/retrieve/pii/S0022202X15370834; http://ieeexplore.ieee.org/document/5288620/.

[22] Aristovich K, Donegá M, Blochet C, et al. Imaging fast neural traffic at fascicular level with electrical impedance tomography: proof of principle in rat sciatic nerve. Journal of Neural Engineering. 2018;15(5):056025.

[23] Rossini PM, Micera S, Benvenuto A, et al. Double nerve intraneural interface implant on a human amputee for robotic hand control. Clinical Neurophysiology. 2010;121(5):777–783. Available from: http://dx.doi.org/10.1016/j.clinph.2010.01.001.

[24] Micera S, Rossini PM, Rigosa J, et al. Decoding of grasping information from neural signals recorded using peripheral intrafascicular interfaces. Journal of NeuroEngineering and Rehabilitation. 2011;8(1):2–11.

[25] Clark GA, Wendelken S, Page DM, et al. Using multiple high-count electrode arrays in human median and ulnar nerves to restore sensorimotor function after previous transradial amputation of the hand. In: 2014 36th Annual International Conference of the IEEE Engineering in Medicine and Biology Society, EMBC 2014; 2014. p. 1977–1980.

[26] Schultz AE and Kuiken TA. Neural interfaces for control of upper limb prostheses: the state of the art and future possibilities. PM and R. 2011;3(1): 55–67.

[27] Brindley GS, Polkey CE, and Rushton DN. Sacral anterior root stimulators for bladder control in paraplegia. Paraplegia. 1982;20(6):365–381. Available from: http://www.pubmedcentral.nih.gov/articlerender.fcgi?artid= 1029041&tool=pmcentrez&rendertype=abstract.

[28] Mortimer JT and Bhadra N. Fundamentals of Electrical Stimulation. 2nd ed. Elsevier Ltd; 2018. Available from: https://doi.org/10.1016/ B978-0-12-805353-9.00006-1.

[29] Cutrone A and Micera S. Implantable neural interfaces and wearable tactile systems for bidirectional neuroprosthetics systems. Advanced Healthcare Materials. 2019;8:1801345. Available from: https://onlinelibrary.wiley.com/ doi/abs/10.1002/adhm.201801345.

[30] Wongsarnpigoon A and Grill WM. Energy-efficient waveform shapes for neural stimulation revealed with a genetic algorithm. Journal of Neural Engineering. 2010;7(4):046009. Available from: http://stacks.iop.org/1741-2552/ 7/i=4/a=046009?key=crossref.b2a503428f3820e6d2994c496acc3d4.

[31] Pasluosta C, Kiele P, and Stieglitz T. Paradigms for restoration of somatosensory feedback via stimulation of the peripheral nervous system. Clinical Neurophysiology. 2018;129(4):851–862. Available from: https://doi.org/10. 1016/j.clinph.2017.12.027.

[32] Shannon RV. A model of safe levels for electrical stimulation. IEEE Transactions on Biomedical Engineering. 1992;39(4):424–426. Available from: http://ieeexplore.ieee.org/document/126616/.

[33] Grill WM. Waveforms for Neural Stimulation. 2nd ed. Elsevier Ltd; 2018. Available from: https://doi.org/10.1016/B978-0-12-805353-9.00008-5.

[34] Clippinger FW, Avery R, and Titus BR. Sensory feedback system for an upper-limb amputation prosthesis. Bulletin of Prosthetics Research. 1974: 247–258.

[35] Brunton E, Silveira C, Rosenberg J, Schiefer M, Riddell J, and Nazarpour K. Temporal modulation of the response of sensory fibers to paired-pulse stimulation. IEEE Transactions on Neural Systems and Rehabilitation Engineering. 2019;27(9):1676–1683.

[36] Raspopovic S, Capogrosso M, Petrini FM, *et al.* Bioengineering: restoring natural sensory feedback in real-time bidirectional hand prostheses. Science Translational Medicine. 2014;6(222):1–12.

[37] Tan DW, Schiefer MA, Keith MW, Anderson JR, Tyler J, and Tyler DJ. A neural interface provides long-term stable natural touch perception. Science Translational Medicine. 2014;6(257):257ra138.

[38] Schiefer M, Tan D, Sidek SM, and Tyler DJ. Sensory feedback by peripheral nerve stimulation improves task performance in individuals with upper limb loss using a myoelectric prosthesis. Journal of Neural Engineering. 2015;13(1):016001.

[39] Ortiz-Catalan M, Hakansson B, and Branemark R. An osseointegrated human-machine gateway for long-term sensory feedback and motor control of artificial limbs. Science Translational Medicine. 2014;6(257):257re6.

[40] Gaunt RA, Hokanson JA, and Weber DJ. Microstimulation of primary afferent neurons in the L7 dorsal root ganglia using multielectrode arrays in anesthetized cats: thresholds and recruitment properties. Journal of Neural Engineering. 2009;6(5):055009.

[41] Brindley GS. The first 500 patients with sacral anterior root stimulator implants: general description. Spinal Cord. 1994;32(12):795–805.

[42] Kandel ER, Schwartz J. Principles of Neural Science. 5th ed. McGraw-Hill Publishing; 2012.

[43] Okorokova EV, He Q, and Bensmaia SJ. Biomimetic encoding model for restoring touch in bionic hands through a nerve interface. Journal of Neural Engineering. 2018;15(6):066033.

[44] Saal HP, Delhaye BP, Rayhaun BC, and Bensmaia SJ. Simulating tactile signals from the whole hand with millisecond precision. Proceedings of the National Academy of Sciences of the United States of America. 2017;114(28):E5693–E5702.

[45] Valle G, Mazzoni A, Iberite F, *et al.* Biomimetic intraneural sensory feedback enhances sensation naturalness, tactile sensitivity, and manual dexterity in a bidirectional prosthesis. Neuron. 2018;100(1):37–45. Available from: https://doi.org/10.1016/j.neuron.2018.08.033.

[46] Kuiken TA, Miller LA, Lipschutz RD, *et al.* Targeted reinnervation for enhanced prosthetic arm function in a woman with a proximal amputation: a case study. Lancet. 2007;369(9559):371–380.

[47] Wendelken S, Page DM, Davis T, *et al.* Restoration of motor control and proprioceptive and cutaneous sensation in humans with prior upper-limb amputation via multiple Utah Slanted Electrode Arrays (USEAs) implanted in residual peripheral arm nerves. Journal of NeuroEngineering and Rehabilitation. 2017;14(1):1–17.

Chapter 7

Surgical considerations for advanced prosthetic control and residual limb pain management in amputees

Aidan Roche[1,2]

Amputations are typically more common in the lower limb due to diabetes and vascular disease than the upper limb, where the leading aetiology is trauma, although this does vary between developed and developing countries [1,2]. In both situations, traditional surgical teaching has focused on leaving enough soft tissue to cover the residual bone for comfortable prosthetic fitting [3]. Involved nerves are usually cut under tension, so that the nerve stump becomes buried under muscular soft tissue to prevent painful neuromas at the amputation site itself, which will prevent comfortable socket fitting. However, with advances in secondary surgical procedures following amputation, new evidence is suggesting that nerve transfers may prevent resulting pain symptoms [4].

The surgical management of patients following an amputation can be guided by the level, functional requirement and pain symptoms of the patient [5]. For some patients, the initial trauma and resulting amputation surgery are enough, and patients do not want further surgery even if functional and analgesic benefits could be provided to them. This naturally should be respected after careful discussion of the options available to them, and onward referral to rehabilitation and pain team management should be made.

In patients who are seeking treatment to improve prosthetic control and/or relieve phantom/residual limb pain, there are surgical options available based on the level of the amputation. In transradial patients, whether unilateral or bilateral, advances in signal processing which provide simultaneous and proportional control mean that surface EMG-controlled prostheses should be sufficient for most activities of daily living [6,7]. It should be noted that hand dominance will transfer to the contralateral, remaining limb.

For higher-level amputations, either transhumeral or glenohumeral, targeted muscle reinnervation (TMR) has proven to be an effective technique to provide simultaneous control of multiple degrees of freedom at the elbow, wrist and hand [8,9].

[1]The University of Edinburgh, Edinburgh, UK
[2]Department of Plastic Surgery, NHS Lothian, Edinburgh, UK

TMR is a nerve transfer technique where amputated nerves which once had distal muscular targets can be rerouted to proximal muscles, which no longer have functional benefit due to the amputation. For example, in the case of a glenohumeral amputee, as the arm has been amputated, the pectoral muscles (major and minor) have lost their main functions. As such, these healthy muscles can be used for more important functions such as opening or closing a prosthetic hand through signal processing and training the patient. This is achieved by denervating these proximal muscles of their original nerve supply and coapting the chosen distal nerve to the transection point. Potential nerve transfer matrices have previously been documented, and these should be tailored to each patient's unique anatomy following trauma and any previous reconstructive attempts [10]. Using existing proportional surface EMG electrodes which are widely available in clinical practice, up to 6–7 degrees of freedom can be simultaneously controlled in this manner. Higher degrees of freedom can be achieved with high density electrode arrays, but this remains limited to the research arena and has yet to make it to clinical practice [11].

One of the main benefits of TMR, which has been realised through increased numbers of patients undergoing this procedure, is the relief of previously untreatable neuroma, residual and phantom limb pain [12]. This has been confirmed in randomised control trials against standard medical treatment and should be considered in all patients who have ongoing pain symptoms [4]. Such is the relief of pain symptoms that some patients elect to undergo TMR purely for this benefit as opposed to prosthetic control [10].

While TMR has become a clinically accepted treatment option, further surgical innovations are being developed to further refine the feedforward and feedback arms of the control loop. Regenerative peripheral nerve interfaces (RPNIs) use smaller muscle grafts innervated either by the transected peripheral nerve or by individual fascicles of that nerve to increase the signal-to-noise ratio for more precise control of individual movements with reduced need for complex signal processing [13]. Much like TMR, RPNIs act as biological amplifiers of peripheral nerve's efferent signals but differ as they can allow more discrete movements such as individual finger flexion. Similar to TMR, early evidence suggests that RPNIs provide relief of residual limb, neuroma and phantom limb pain but further randomised control trials are needed to substantiate these promising results [14].

In situations where there is insufficient remnant muscle in the residual limb for basic prosthetic control, autologous and innervated muscle can be transferred from other regions of the patient's body. By building on the concept of free functioning muscle transfer, bionic reconstruction allows the creation of new neuromuscular interfaces that can amplify the desired physiological signals. This has been shown to work not just in patients with mangled or burnt limbs, but also in patients who have sustained avulsion injuries of their brachial plexus resulting in an insensate and functionless limb [14,15]. By demonstrating to the patients that they can regain control of prosthetic hand, in some cases many decades after their original injuries, they are able to electively choose amputation of a useless limb in favour of a more functional prosthesis.

Alongside the previous concepts, implantable myoelectric sensors (IMES) have been developed to increase the accuracy of prosthetic control [16]. By placing IMES directly into the bellies of remnant muscles, the signal-to-noise ratio can be increased, and the intended movements of the user be executed with less errors. This has been demonstrated in both transradial and transhumeral amputees, with increased accuracy when compared to surface myoelectric control [17,18]. The IMES system requires an induction coil to work, so can only be used in residual limbs, and cannot be used in glenohumeral amputees.

Another important consideration, alongside the control architecture, is the manner in which the prosthesis is attached to the patient. For transradial patients, the standard reverse moulding technique to develop a socket is sufficient. There are promising developments in this arena, with new lightweight and breathable fabric sockets being manufactured, which remain strong enough to support a terminal device but are lightweight, comfortable and allow sweating in a more normal fashion. However, for higher amputation levels, external fitting of a socket may not be the most functional. Innovating on known dental practices, where the ability of titanium to bond with bone, in a process known as osseointegration, has enabled several groups to demonstrate that a percutaneous bone implant can safely traverse the soft tissue to suspend a prosthesis [19]. As the prosthesis becomes an extension of the skeleton itself, the weight of the prosthesis is no longer as noticeable to the patient, and they are able to complete greater ranges of motion. A good example of this is the transhumeral amputee being able to reach easily above their head with their prosthesis, a task which is very difficult for socket-wearing users.

The main concern with osseointegration is the increased risk of infection around the percutaneous site, and whether skin infections could migrate to the bone leading to osteomyelitis and ultimately implant failure [20]. A novel technique that has been developed to overcome this while taking advantage of skeletal support is the use of a reversed T-shaped implant, whose edges mimic those of the condyles of bone thereby acting as a support for an external socket [21].

When patients are asked what function they would most like enabled in their prostheses, the return of sensation is high on that priority list. Understandably, this has been a more challenging problem to solve surgically, as sensation is not limited to fine touch, but vibration, proprioception, heat and pain. Each has their own pathway in the peripheral nervous system, and accurately stimulating those pathways will be of most use to the amputees themselves. Non-invasive systems have been trialled in research laboratories with various forms of haptic or electrotactile feedback, but these are yet to make their way to clinical applications [22].

Invasive feedback systems have begun to explore the use of different implantable electrodes that interface with peripheral nerves in some manner. Electrodes that have been implanted into the nerves have been demonstrated to return the sensation of touch in patients while controlling a prosthetic hand [23,24]. Although these studies are encouraging, concerns remain regarding the damage to the intraneural tissue from direct implantation and loss of signal quality over time as scar tissue forms. Other groups have used cuff electrodes to stimulate this effect and have developed home trial systems to determine the long-term efficacy of these systems [25,26].

Osseointegration has also been used to provide a gateway for bidirectional interfacing with peripheral nerves and may prove to be useful in higher-level amputees [27]. Study participants who have used these systems have been reported to embody their prosthesis more, one of the hurdles necessary to overcome for long-term adoption of prosthetic technology.

One of the more difficult sensations to replicate is proprioception, or the awareness of joint position in space. For example, when you move your hand with your eyes closed, you are aware of where your hand is in relation to your body. One approach to addressing this deficit is the creation of an agonist–antagonist myoneural interface, where remnant opposing muscles are connected to each other. When one muscle contracts, it stretches the other, activating mechanoreceptors within the muscle and enabling the patient to gain proprioceptive information. When coupled with a 2 degree of freedom prosthetic ankle in a transtibial amputee, improved prosthetic control was noted when compared to amputees with standard surgical amputations [28,29].

Altogether, these promising surgical interventions can provide more function for amputees and address residual pain symptoms which are intractable to current medical management. While each of these techniques addresses individual aspects of limb loss, none have totally addressed all the factors necessary to replace a natural limb. Indeed, the combination of one or more of these techniques may be additive, resulting in a sum which is greater than its individual parts. Encouragingly, current combinations of bioengineering and surgical methods are at least equivalent to hand transplantation, without the side effects of immunosuppression and increased skin cancer risks and lifelong medications nor rely on a donor to provide a limb [30]. As technology continues to improve, surgical techniques will evolve to adapt to innovations resulting in better outcomes for patients.

References

[1]   Varma P, Stineman MG, and Dillingham TR. Epidemiology of limb loss. Physical Medicine and Rehabilitation Clinics of North America. 2014;25(1):1–8.

[2]   Bibi R, Kamran B, Minhas MA, and Siddiqui NY. Epidemiology of amputation. The Professional Medical Journal. 2007;20(2):261–265.

[3]   Persson B. Lower limb amputation Part 1: Amputation methods – a 10 year literature review. Prosthetics and Orthotics International. 2001;25(1):7–13.

[4]   Dumanian GA, Potter BK, Mioton LM, *et al.* Targeted muscle reinnervation treats neuroma and phantom pain in major limb amputees. Annals of Surgery. 2019;270(2):238–246.

[5]   Roche AD, Lakey B, Mendez I, Vujaklija I, Farina D, and Aszmann OC. Clinical perspectives in upper limb prostheses: An update. Current Surgery Reports. 2019;7(3):5.

[6]   Amsuess S, Vujaklija I, Goebel P, *et al.* Context-dependent upper limb prosthesis control for natural and robust use. IEEE Transactions on Neural Systems and Rehabilitation Engineering. 2016;24(7):744–753.

[7]   Krasoulis A, Vijayakumar S, and Nazarpour K. Multi-grip classification-based prosthesis control with two EMG-IMU sensors. IEEE Transactions on Neural Systems and Rehabilitation Engineering. 2020;28(2):508–518.

[8]   Kuiken TA, Childress DS, and Rymer WZ. The hyper-reinnervation of rat skeletal muscle. Brain Research. 1995;676(1):113–123.

[9]   Kuiken TA, Li G, Lock BA, *et al.* Targeted muscle reinnervation for real-time myoelectric control of multifunction artificial arms. JAMA. 2009;301(6): 619–628.

[10]   Salminger S, Sturma A, Roche AD, Mayer JA, Gstoettner C, and Aszmann OC. Outcomes, challenges, and pitfalls after targeted muscle reinnervation in high-level amputees. Plastic and Reconstructive Surgery. 2019;144(6):1037e–1043e.

[11]   Kapelner T, Jiang N, Holobar A, *et al.* Motor unit characteristics after targeted muscle reinnervation. PLoS One. 2016;11(2):1–12. Available from: https://doi.org/10.1371/journal.pone.0149772.

[12]   McNamara CT and Iorio ML. Targeted muscle reinnervation: Outcomes in treating chronic pain secondary to extremity amputation and phantom limb syndrome. Journal of Reconstructive Microsurgery. 2020;36(4):235–240.

[13]   Vu PP, Vaskov AK, Irwin ZT, *et al.* A regenerative peripheral nerve interface allows real-time control of an artificial hand in upper limb amputees. Science Translational Medicine. 2020;12(533):eaay2857.

[14]   Kubiak CA, Kemp SWP, and Cederna PS. Regenerative peripheral nerve interface for management of postamputation neuroma. JAMA Surgery. 2018;153(7):681–682.

[15]   Vujaklija OCAI, Roche AD, Salminger S, *et al.* Elective amputation and bionic substitution restore functional hand use after critical soft tissue injuries. Scientific Reports. 2016;6:34960.

[16]   Weir RFF, Troyk PR, DeMichele G, and Kuiken T. Implantable myoelectric sensors (IMES) for upper-extremity prosthesis control – preliminary work. In: Proceedings of the 25th Annual International Conference of the IEEE Engineering in Medicine and Biology Society (EMBC). vol. 2; 2003. p. 1562–1565.

[17]   Pasquina PF, Evangelista M, Carvalho AJ, *et al.* First-in-man demonstration of a fully implanted myoelectric sensors system to control an advanced electromechanical prosthetic hand. Journal of Neuroscience Methods. 2015;244: 85–93.

[18]   Salminger S, Sturma A, Hofer C, *et al.* Long-term implant of intramuscular sensors and nerve transfers for wireless control of robotic arms in above-elbow amputees. Science Robotics. 2019;4(32):eaaw6306.

[19]   Jönsson S, Caine-Winterberger K, and Brånemark R. Osseointegration amputation prostheses on the upper limbs: Methods, prosthetics and rehabilitation. Prosthetics and Orthotics International. 2011;35(2):190–200.

[20]   Hebert JS, Rehani M, and Stiegelmar R. Osseointegration for lower-limb amputation. JBJS Reviews. 2017;5(10):e10.

[21]   Salminger S, Gradischar A, Skiera R, *et al.* Attachment of upper arm prostheses with a subcutaneous osseointegrated implant in transhumeral amputees. Prosthetics and Orthotics International. 2018;42(1):93–100.

[22]   Wilke M, Hartmann C, Schimpf F, Farina D, and Dosen S. The interaction between feedback type and learning in routine grasping with myoelectric prostheses. IEEE Transactions on Haptics. 2020;13(3):645–654

[23]   Rossini PM, Micera S, Benvenuto A, *et al.* Double nerve intraneural interface implant on a human amputee for robotic hand control. Clinical Neurophysiology. 2010;121(5):777–783.

[24]   Raspopovic S, Capogrosso M, Petrini FM, *et al.* Restoring natural sensory feedback in real-time bidirectional hand prostheses. Science Translational Medicine. 2014;6(222):222ra19.

[25]   Dhillon GS, Lawrence SM, Hutchinson DT, and Horch KW. Residual function in peripheral nerve stumps of amputees: Implications for neural control of artificial limbs. The Journal of Hand Surgery. 2004;29(4):605–615.

[26]   Tan DW, Schiefer MA, Keith MW, Anderson JR, Tyler J, and Tyler DJ. A neural interface provides long-term stable natural touch perception. Science Translational Medicine. 2014;6(257):257ra138.

[27]   Ortiz-Catalan M, Brånemark EMR, and Håkansson B. Direct neural sensory feedback and control via osseointegration. In: XVI World Congress of the International Society for Prosthetics and Orthotics (ISPO); 2017. p. 1–2.

[28]   Srinivasan SS, Carty MJ, Calvaresi PW, *et al.* On prosthetic control: A regenerative agonist-antagonist myoneural interface. Science Robotics. 2017;2(6):eaan2971.

[29]   Clites TR, Carty MJ, Ullauri JB, *et al.* Proprioception from a neurally controlled lower-extremity prosthesis. Science Translational Medicine. 2018;10(443):eaap8373.

[30]   Salminger S, Sturma A, Roche AD, *et al.* Functional and psychosocial outcomes of hand transplantation compared with prosthetic fitting in below-elbow amputees: A multicenter cohort study. PLoS One. 2016;11(9):1–13.

Chapter 8
User-prosthesis coadaptation

Carles Igual[1], Jorge Igual[1], Janne Hahne[2]
and Kianoush Nazarpour[3]

In the early stages of myoelectric control for upper limb prostheses, researchers focused on obtaining the most optimal model for the prosthesis control (Figure 8.1) [1–6]. The focus was on the fast growing machine-learning field, where a wide range of potential methods were available. Having already developed machine-learning models in other areas leads to an accelerated evolution of the research in prosthetics. A broad variety of algorithms were applied to estimate the user's intent in upper limb movements among others. High-performance models were generated facing the task with completely different perspectives not finding a unique solution for the problem [7–9]. Despite these promising results and the newer developments of more complex and powerful algorithms, the older and simpler models remained as the main option for the prostheses control. A clear example of this is the most commonly used control protocol for commercial prosthesis: a basic one degree of freedom (DoF) control switching system. The machine-learning developments have so far not succeeded to replace the conventional 2-channel systems in a large scale. Even if these approaches presented an excellent behavior in controlled and specific environments, migrating to the real world has become a challenging task. In daily use, reliability of machine-learning modes remains an issue and regular recalibration may be required for some users. These first approaches were considering the machine as the only agent that could learn. But the machine's learning is not the only factor that can be used to improve the overall system's performance, the user's learning can be integrated too.

Originally, the models were mainly developed via off-line investigations [10–13]. The data was previously recorded and then the model was trained and tested in an off-line scenario. The machine and the participant did not interact in those phases. The two agents of the process were completely separated. Later on, the researchers realized that while testing the algorithms on-line [14], the users were able to correct behaviors where the machine was failing in the off-line evaluation. The reason on-line tests were outperforming off-line protocols was the human adaptation [15–25]. The

[1]Universitat Politècnica de València, València, Spain
[2]University Medical Center Göttingen, Göttingen, Germany
[3]The University of Edinburgh, Edinburgh, UK

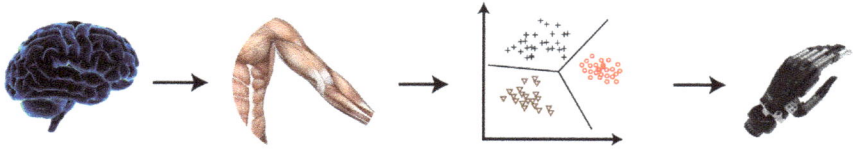

Figure 8.1   *Generic prosthesis control scheme. The human patterns are used as*
input (in this case EMG signals extracted form an armband) by the
machine to estimate an output (applied to a prosthesis or in a virtual
environment) of the user's attempted action

human modified their behavior to compensate errors induced by the machine or by external perturbation. Because of the real-time feedback, the user could adapt to the machine's behaviour. From here, human adaptation has been considered an essential element of the closed-loop structure learning and a powerful tool for improving the system's performance. Two learners were participating in the learning process: the machine and the human. The common, but not necessary, way to make the user interact with the machine was during the test phase once the model was learned. All along the learning process the user and the machine remained separated. The users were meant to perform the requested signals during a data acquisition period. Afterward, the machine was being trained with the recorded data. The user did not play any active role in the process of learning the model and that was only machine learning. Human learning was adapting the human behavior to the previously learned model with the goal of achieving the highest performance possible during the test. On-line studies allowed the users to adapt to the systems' output and correct the EMG signals they were generating in order to achieve the desired target. This improved the systems' performance but the gap between the academia and the industry remained significant.

Seeking to boost the benefits of human–machine interaction, some groups tried including the user as an adaptive agent into the model learning phase as well [24,26]. These first trials triggered the concept of coadaptation. The essence is that both agents adapt at the same time with a common goal of helping each other to learn the optimal model. Before getting deeper in the coadaptation benefits, it is necessary to identify the role each learner plays in the learning process so we can understand the interaction between them.

8.1 Machine adaptation

We will focus our attention on the machine's learning process first. The objective for the machine here is to learn the underlying information of the data used as input. Since the beginning, it is necessary to define which kind of information we want the machine to understand and learn. The models are divided into two approaches: classification [7,23,27,28] and regression [9,22,25,29–33]. The difference relies on the system's output: a label to tag the input data in a class (classification) or a continuous mapping

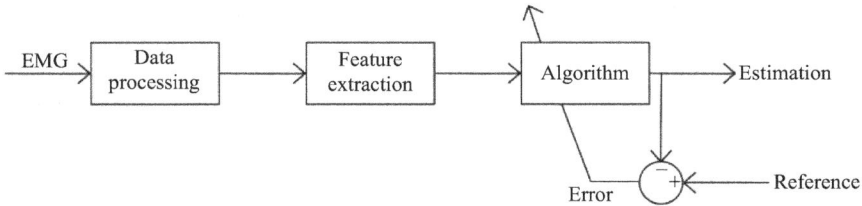

Figure 8.2   Example of a machine-learning process. EMG's signals are used as input for feature extraction. The features are used to train an adaptive model with an error-based cost function

of the output (regression). However, for our interests both approaches follow the same learning procedure.

As it is shown in Figure 8.2, the initial step is to feed the system with the input data that forms the base for the variables the machine should estimate. A proper choice of input variables is crucial for the system's performance. If the data is not appropriate, the machine will not be able to learn what is desired. We will go deeper in this later as it involves the human also. For now, the goal is to understand the learning that both learners go through individually.

Once the data acquisition is complete, features are extracted in a block-wise manner [34]. Features will then be the input for the learning algorithm. Feature extraction isolates meaningful information from the input data and simplifies the learning task for the machine, discarding irrelevant information. The executed patterns should correspond to features as independent as possible for different motions, so the model is capable of differentiating them.

During algorithmic training, the machine receives the data and forms a model to estimate the output. In the case of myoelectric control, this is to extract the user intend from the EMG features. Depending on the complexity of the machine learner, the provided repetitions for each of the contraction patterns need to be consistent within each class and separable across different classes. Similar constraints apply in the case of regression. The number of independent patterns the user is able to generate in a repetitive way determines the maximal number of functions or DoFs that can be controlled.

This could be a limitation for some users because of their limb deficiencies. The physiology of the stump could limit the capability of generating enough EMG patterns [35]. Algorithms that work with multiple DoFs in able-bodied have also to be tested in amputees for this reason. The system's final goal is to achieve a natural and proportional control of multiple DoFs. Usually commercial devices can control only one DoF at a time without any machine-learning program. The selection of the DoF is done with an activation function that allows the user to switch between DoFs. The output value depends on a metric extracted from the EMGs as it could be the amplitude of the signal. Obviously, this mapping is not natural and requires long training sessions for the user to learn how to control the prosthesis. Due to the non-learning protocols, all the adaptation lies on the human. With the newer machine-learning models, it has been tried to learn the underlying correlations between the EMG signals and the movement generated [36]. This gives the prosthesis control a more natural movement and intuitive relation with the signals. The similarities with a real hand are higher, due to the machine's ability to learn. The modeling of EMG-movement relationship helps the user to learn a more intuitive control.

8.2   Human adaptation

Now we will move on to the second agent of the learning process, the human. Humans can adapt their behavior to achieve a better performance. Ison *et al.* [14] studied the human-learning skills and their effects on the final system's performance. Like in every task, the user is able through practice to improve their results with a fixed model [15,21] and become more stable and consistent in the signal generation. Recently, studies focused on finding the right tools to help the user understand the system's output and interact with it. The comprehension of the system would make the human adaptation process more efficient [37]. Complex environments where the user does not understand the given feedback would not allow them to learn and adapt. Because of this, finding the best feedback to exploit the benefits of human adaptation and improving the user experience has gained relevance in recent years.

As expected, the human-learning process seen in prosthesis control follows the stages of a typical motor skill learning for a new task. The first step is to understand the general remit of the task but not necessarily the details. This understanding is achieved through repetition and practice where an appropriate feedback map would play a fundamental role [18,21,24,38]. Finally, once the user builds the appropriate internal model, they can perform the task (in this case controlling the prosthesis) readily. At this point, the user has learned and performs significantly better than during the first trials due to the experience gained. Strazzulla *et al.* [16] proved the hypothesis of how experienced users outperform amateurs. The difference between the two groups was not in the accuracy metric, both were able to complete the task. The difference was on the time metrics, experienced users completed the target faster than amateurs. Their experience made them aware of the shortest strategies to reach the target so they performed it straight way. Opposite to this, the amateurs that did not have any experience had to search for an optimal strategy before executing the task. Being the completion time, the main difference between both groups' performances (and not the completion ratio) made the researchers set the cause in the human adaptation and not the machine-learning process. The larger experience of more experienced users was translated into a more efficient behavior.

The initial idea of taking advantage of human adaptation was conducting an on-line prosthesis control test [39]. The fixed model learned with the user's EMGs is tested in real time, giving the control to the participant. The on-line control with feedback to the human created a closed-loop structure as in Figure 8.3. The feedback of the machine's output could be used by the human to adapt their behavior to the machine improving the system's performance with respect to the previous off-line

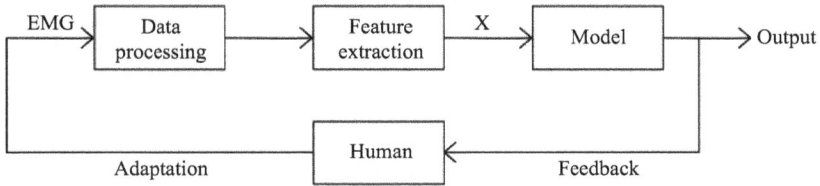

Figure 8.3   Closed-loop structure. The output of the machine generates the input of the human and vice versa

proposals [40,41]. Human adaptation is able to solve some robustness issues that prostheses users were facing in experimental applications due to the nonstationary EMG signals. Due to the given feedback, the user is able to correct their contraction pattern and compensate potential disturbances. This user real-time reaction was tested by Hahne *et al.* [17]. They conducted an experiment adding noise to the EMG signals and testing on-line the capability of the user of maintaining a stable control. The results showed that the noise disturbances were countered successfully. Comparing a classification algorithm against a regression method, the regression had a better performance due to the continuous output. This study proved that with the right feedback, the user can understand the process and adapt properly to unstable situations avoiding degradation in the system's behavior.

8.3   Recalibration

As we have said, sometimes the user is able to counter some undesired effects of the nonstationarities. However, what human adaptation can overcome has its limits and in other occasions the user cannot succeed in dealing with the system's degradation. There can be multiple reasons for a model to stop performing as well as at the beginning: different sensor positioning [42], EMG patterns that are not consistent through time [43,44], the user [45], etc. In these scenarios, the possibility of recalibrating the model is a suitable solution [41].

The idea of recalibration is to retrain the model with new data in order to adapt it to the present, and probably new, conditions. The human is in constant adaptation using the system daily, leading to some modifications in their behavior. The patterns he ends up using could not be the same with the ones used for training the model. After some time, the machine could need to go through an adaptive process if we want the system to stay functional. With recalibration, what we try to achieve is to adapt the machine to the EMGs that the human is using after some time since the model was trained.

During this period, the user has been adapting, while the machine remained invariant (human adaptation). The user has been the one taking all the responsibilities to overcome the possible degradation effects. The prosthesis user wants an easy control, so at some point the user efforts could not be enough to deal with degradation, or simply generate an undesired user experience because the great efforts needed. This is the moment when recalibration should be implemented. We have to be aware that this need could be dependent on the user; if the user is comfortable with the behavior or he prefers to stay with the current model, the recalibration will not be necessary. The process will teach the machine some part of the adaptation the user has gone through and readjust their behavior to the present EMG spectrum input. The machine will now be aware of the new conditions and release the user of the needs to force their behavior to achieve a desired performance. With this, we will be updating the machine learning including in their training data the new user knowledge generated with the adaptation. Both agents have adapted independently in different occasions, and with the recalibration we merge both adaptation processes in one common retraining. This could be seen as restarting the process again, but not from scratch. Now the machine and the user have a lot of experience (the initial training data for the machine and all the user adaptation process for the human). Both have gone through a first adaptation process and the cycle would be repeated; the machine will update their learned model and after that the user would readapt to it. However, these new adaptation phases will be shorter as the new information or changes are less different compared to the initial step. The active learner will become the frozen one when the other agent goes under their adaptation process. The agents will be switching their roles through time as the recalibration phases are executed.

The recalibration process can be executed in a wide range of different protocols (example in Figure 8.4). At the beginning, the first approaches were using a more frequent recalibration [46]. Trying to reduce these times, researchers kept developing new ideas until they reached more efficient paradigms [40,41]. To represent the untrained conditions and add them to the training set, Chen *et al.* [47] proposed a training data set expansion during the test. Once the test data was labeled correctly, it was added to the training data set. This procedure was reinforcing the correct labeled data for each cluster trying to reduce the weight of the data that could be leading to

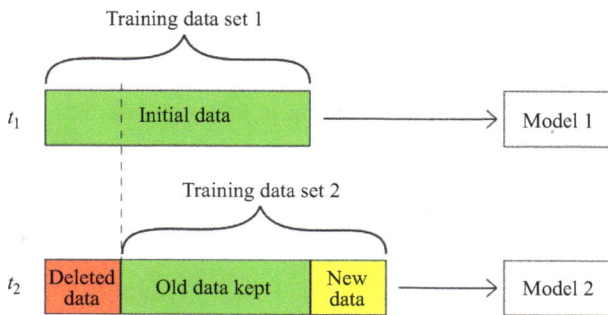

Figure 8.4   Example of a recalibration protocol. Initial data is recorded in t_1 for training the model 1. After some time, in t_2 new data is recorded (yellow). A new training set is configured with the new data and a high percentage of the old data that is kept (green). The oldest (or outdated) data from t_1 will be deleted (red)

misclassification. Expanding the training set proved to have benefits against shorter data sets, so the idea was to increase it with the test data and recalibrate the system with the expanded training set. Yeung *et al.* [48] proposed a similar method but with a directional paradigm. As newer data was being added to the training set, and older data with similar information was being erased. With this, they reduced the distortion to each region generated by redundant and outdated data while updating the training set. The data erased was obsolete as the newer data represented the same condition in a recent situation. The model was receiving the new data representing something already learned that had undergone some small changes. These small changes could not be a problem yet, but in the long run it could end in a poor performance. With recalibration, we are looking to update the system to the present and forget about the past representations.

What all methods have in common is the general concept of recalibration, adding new data to the training set and updating the model to the newest EMG patterns and disturbances. However, it would be ideal that the system does not need recalibration at all [49]. The system should be robust enough to deal with disturbances from the outside and keep their performance stable. The user also does not want to spend their time recalibrating the system very often. Therefore, the recalibration process has to be as fast as possible and requires less time as possible to be usable.

While researchers experimented with recalibration, based on this, the concept of transfer learning emerged [50,51]. The basic concept of transfer learning is that the outdated data (and model) from a task is still usable to update the model to a current state. Because the differences between the past and the present will be small and the basic information carried by the EMG patterns are the same; only a small amount of data will be necessary to update the small changes in the task through time. In this case, we are retraining the model in the same task but in different times succeeding in keeping the high performance. Moreover, researchers found out that the task does not need to be the same to take advantage of previously recorded data. There is underlying information that is shared among similar tasks [52]. This is similar to the idea of structural learning in the motor control community. Structural learning advocates that humans can learn the general structures of a task and then generalize it to other tasks that are related in some base level. So instead of recalibrating for the same function, we could use a similar protocol to learn a new task faster. If there are similar tasks, we could use the data and the model of the previously learned one to learn a new task adding only a small amount of data that represents the differences and updating the previous model. Paaßen *et al.* [51] used this concept to adapt an old myoelectric control model to a new situation where the data was completely obsolete.

8.4   Coadaptive prosthesis control

Now as we studied both the learners, we can look for the opportunities to combine their adaptation processes in one. In the on-line tests, the human is able to adapt their behavior with the objective of reducing the difference between the estimated and the desired output. The human has the opportunity to interact with the machine to achieve the best possible performance. However, in this phase the machine is fixed, it is not adapting, and all the adaptation is being performed by the user. The on-line condition during the test gave the user the possibility of adapting, while the machine had adapted during the model training. The first natural approach for coadaptive systems was to merge both concepts in one, a complete on-line experimentation (training and test) [44,53]. The model is trained at the same time the data is collected, all executed in real time. This closed-loop learning structure gives the two learners, user and machine, influence over the other's learning. This was the beginning of coadaptive systems.

Before coadaptive models, it was obvious that both agents were going through a learning process but separately. Besides, they were learning for their own interest. The data from the other agent was being used as input to adapt and perform as good as possible without considering the other's adaptation process. With the new proposal, the learning becomes cooperative. The coadaptive training makes both agents focus on the same goal: to optimize the model. However, for that purpose they have to take into account all the variables and an important one is the other agent adaptation. Now that both agents adapt at the same time, each of them can react in real time to the other's adaptation and its consequences. So, instead of having one agent learning while the other is off, here both do not have just to adapt to the previously learned situation but also adapt to the new behaviors the other part is adopting. This procedure allowed simpler algorithms to obtain a higher performance avoiding some problems that are present with off-line training [26].

The coadaptation inkling is the common goal for both the learners. The essence is making them work together in order to learn the best model [54]. The novelty relies in that each part does not only adapt to different situations with a prefixed answer. Now the other part adaptation has to be taken into account, too. So, for adapting you do not only have to think in how you should react to an undesired performance but you also have to consider how the other will echo to your new reaction because their behavior is not fixed. The human learning shapes the machine's behavior and vice versa.

The feedback has a great importance in the human learning [30], but it acquires a higher impact in coadaptive systems. The channels of information between human and machine have to send clear information to the receiver about the transmitter actions. The EMG patterns, which would be used by the machine as input, have to be consistent. The same targets need to have similar EMG patterns for the model to be robust. At the same time, the displayed output of the machine has to be clear for the user as it would be their input data for the adaptive process. If the user does not understand the meaning of the feedback, he would not be able to perform consistent EMG patterns or the required correction. Their misunderstanding of the information would probably lead to a poor model with an undesired behavior. Because of the on-line training and the real-time adaptation of both the learners, their inputs would be constantly adapting as well as their outputs. The adaptation of one side will be the input for the adaptation on the other side. This potential continuous adaptation was ignored for a long time in the prostheses control research.

The two-learners problem was modeled by Müller *et al.* [54]. The model describes that the system has two channels of information as in Figure 8.5. The first one goes from the human to the machine. The human sends the myoelectric signals that the machine would take as representation of the user's intent. This channel (human–machine) was developed widely with the evolution of the machine-learning algorithms as we commented earlier. The objective is to decode the encoded information in the EMGs through the machine-learning process. The second channel goes the other way around, from the machine to the user. Here is where the feedback system plays its part. The human would receive a representation of the machine's output through this channel that represents the machine's estimation of the user's intent. This feedback is meant to provide the user data to make him aware of the machine's behavior. The user has an expectation of the machine's behavior, so with the feedback they can evaluate whether there is a need for adaptation or not. The understanding of this data would provide the user the knowledge to change their own behavior in order to correct the possible undesired actions. In the end, both channels could be represented by learning coefficients that would define the system's performance. Both the adaptation processes have an effect on the general cost function. The first experiments showed promising results for prostheses control [26,55]. With coadaptive algorithms, the user will try to minimize the error adapting himself with the real-time feedback they are receiving about what the machine is understanding of what they are attempting. With this information, they can search for the signals that generate the desired output. At the same time, the machine knows what the target is and which EMGs the user is generating so it will adapt its coefficients to get closer to the target with those EMGs. This coadaptive process will continue through the whole training. Once the training is over, the system will have converged to a common solution between the two agents. With this paradigm and interaction, when one of the sides is converging to a local minimum, the other side adaptation could force to avoid this situation and keep searching for a better solution. If the user is not contented with the machine model, they will keep varying the inputs trying to make the machine react and achieve a better performance. The novelty is that instead of a two-phase process, now those coefficients are updated at the same time in one phase. Therefore, the evolution of the cost function would be different than in a two-step paradigm leading to different solutions.

For all these reasons, the experimentation shifted from off-line to on-line. Two on-line phases, training and test, have proven their benefits achieving an optimal model. For coadaptive systems, the training is mainly on-line. The real-time reactions allowed in on-line experimentation would lead to faster adaptive systems with simpler models performing with high accuracy.

An example of this is the work of Igual *et al.* [55], which uses the described closed-loop structure. The study proposed a novel coadaptation strategy with some real-time visual feedback. The real-time feedback allows the user to follow the progress of the training and adapt to it before the model is fixed. The model is based on a linear regression algorithm that is learned, while the user learns to use the system at the same time. This paradigm presented great results in able-bodied and in users with

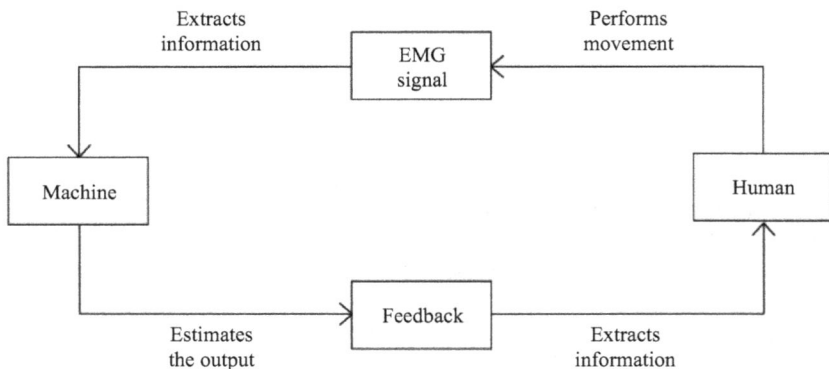

Figure 8.5 Coadaptation scheme. The human receives the machines out through some sort of feedback (sensor, visual or a prosthesis) and reacts according to the feedback. They will generate the desired EMG patterns to achieve the target and send them to the machine

congenital limb deficiency. The on-line training interface allowed the users to generate consistently combined movements, which is a very challenging task for people that lack the natural feedback of an actual limb. Their high performance was comparable to able-bodied people, which has an advantage with the hand natural feedback. The coadaptive system overcame a strong barrier that user with limb deficiency usually has using more developed algorithms that include multiple DoFs. It is not easy for them to generate combined movements without any kind of feedback that allows them to reproduce the pattern consistently. Also it can be stated that the coadaptive learning allowed a simple regression model to outperform the state-of-the-art regression controls. As a result of coadaptive learning and the simplicity of the algorithm, the computational time was reduced compared to more complex state-of-the-art methods. During the experimentation, the researchers noticed that, in situations where off-line training could have led to undesired solutions, the human forced other strategies to generate the right patterns until the machine reacted.

Couraud *et al.* [56] also studied the effects of coadaptation in the field of myoelectric control. They designed a model of human adaptation and performed different levels of coadaptation. With a gain parameter (with a value of 1 as fast human adaptation) they controlled the speed of the human model adaptation to the data. Low adaptation gain values generated a model too slow to perform a full adaptation and high values were too unstable to adapt to the added noise. At the end, the best solution was a variable gain system combining the benefits of both.

8.5 Conclusion

As we have seen, there are two potential learners in machine-learning-based prosthesis control systems. Depending on the structure defined for the control loop, the adaptation process will differ. The machine-learning process has been exploited since the introduction of it to this field. However, the human–machine adaptation was not as important as it is now. In the most recent studies, the human adaptation has shown significant influence in the system's performance and a great potential to be used as a solution to the most common obstacles. In these scenarios, coadaptive systems raise as an option to take advantage of maximizing the benefits of both adaptation processes to overcome the difficulties. The coadaptation idea lies in making the human and the machine learn simultaneously and dependently on the other's learning. These coadaptive implementations have already allowed simple algorithms to present a robust and high performance against disturbances solving some of the most common problems among prostheses control algorithms. However, the commercial prostheses are still majorly controlled by old non-learning control protocols that do not allow the user to have a natural control of the hand. The reason is that these simple and old paradigms are still the most robust option. The academia has made great advances in the prostheses control algorithms, but the achievements have been only partly transferred into the industry. However, the research has shifted from very controlled environments to more realistic conditions, which points the future research path. It is clear that the current goal is to improve the user experience. Advanced algorithms have been already developed with high performances. The challenge is to transfer these algorithms into real scenarios, reaching stable conditions in daily life. Here is where coadaptive models could be a solution to the gap between the academia and the industry and one step toward a solution.

The most important element in a real scenario are the users. At the end, they are the ones who will utilize the system, and their interests and opinions have to be taken into account. This is why the research is more focused in reaching the user than before. Having a high accuracy could not be as valuable as having a good user experience. That is one of the reasons why studies shifted to a more realistic experimentation trying to evaluate the real usability. The coadaptation concept has the advantage that it incorporates the user in the training process and generates a shared experience between user and machine. The theoretical benefits of the coadaptation systems have been already explained. But there are some qualitative benefits that the user experiences too. The process is now more personal and the user can feel how the machine learns with him. This relation makes the control more natural and intuitive as it is more similar to how humans learn to use their bodies. The idea at the end is to have a prosthesis that feels as similar as possible as a real hand. For this, it seems natural to involve the user as much as the machine during the training of the hand. This will help the user to feel the control protocol as theirs and not as an external forced model. There are other reasons for the studies to shift to a more realistic experimentation, other elements that will be relevant for improving the user experience. The robustness of the prosthesis control is a clue element in the future of the field. A prosthesis has to be robust, not just to reach the market but also to have a high acceptance among the users. Users with limb deficiencies would rather not use a prosthesis and overcome their necessities in another way than using a prosthesis that does not make their lives easier. The ideal situation would be where the prosthesis reaction is always the one expected by the user.

The system has to have a robust behavior against the different disturbances the user will face during the time they are using the prosthesis. The electrodes will not be always placed in the same location, the EMG patterns will change for the same movement depending on the arm position, fatigue or other external conditions will affect the system. The prosthesis cannot have an erratic behavior depending on external states unavoidable for the user. Thus, an optimal system should be usable in almost all common conditions with a high performance and not only in controlled environments. At the same time, the easy use of the prosthesis is also important. Tedious training protocols and complicated control structures, in order to achieve a robust performance, are not a solution and will lead to rejection. The use of a prosthesis has to be intuitive and natural, and for this a clear communication between the two agents is essential. Here the training paradigms play a key role and researchers will have to give them the attention proportional to their high relevance in the final outcome. For this, it is essential that the training procedures are clear for the user so the learned model is consistent. Coadaptive models are potential candidates to achieve these requisites. So the model is shaped by the user's learning and therefore by their comprehension of the system. These models will be then more logical for the own user and adapted to their way of understanding the control, increasing the final usability.

References

[1]   Karlik B, Tokhi MO, and Alci M. A fuzzy clustering neural network architecture for multifunction upper-limb prosthesis. IEEE Transactions on Biomedical Engineering. 2003;50(11):1255–1261.

[2]   Kelly MF, Parker PA, and Scott RN. The application of neural networks to myoelectric signal analysis: A preliminary study. IEEE Transactions on Biomedical Engineering. 1990;37(3):221–230.

[3]   Englehart K, Hudgins B. A robust, real-time control scheme for multifunction myoelectric control. IEEE Transactions on Biomedical Engineering. 2003;50(7):848–854.

[4]   Parker P, Englehart K, and Hudgins B. Myoelectric signal processing for control of powered limb prostheses. Journal of Electromyography and Kinesiology. 2006;16(6):541–548.

[5]   Huang Y, Englehart KB, Hudgins B, and Chan AD. A Gaussian mixture model based classification scheme for myoelectric control of powered upper limb prostheses. IEEE Transactions on Biomedical Engineering. 2005;52(11):1801–1811.

[6]   Nazarpour K, Cipriani C, Farina D, and Kuiken T. Guest Editorial: Advances in control of multi-functional powered upper-limb prostheses. IEEE Transactions on Neural Systems and Rehabilitation Engineering. 2014;22(4):711–715.

[7]   Castellini C and van der Smagt P. Surface EMG in advanced hand prosthetics. Biological Cybernetics. 2009;100(1):35–47.

[8] Ameri A, Kamavuako EN, Scheme EJ, Englehart KB, and Parker PA. Real-time, simultaneous myoelectric control using visual target-based training paradigm. Biomedical Signal Processing and Control. 2014;13:8–14.

[9] Hochberg LR, Serruya MD, Friehs GM, *et al.* Neuronal ensemble control of prosthetic devices by a human with tetraplegia. Nature. 2006;442(7099):164.

[10] Nazarpour K, Sharafat AR, and Firoozabadi SM. Application of higher order statistics to surface electromyogram signal classification. IEEE Transactions on Biomedical Engineering. 2007;54(10):1762–1769.

[11] Jiang N, Englehart KB, and Parker PA. Extracting simultaneous and proportional neural control information for multiple-DOF prostheses from the surface electromyographic signal. IEEE Transactions on Bio-Medical Engineering. 2009;56(4):1070–1080.

[12] Hahne JM, Rehbaum H, Biessmann F, *et al.* Simultaneous and proportional control of 2D wrist movements with myoelectric signals. In: 2012 IEEE International Workshop on Machine Learning for Signal Processing; 2012 Sep. p. 1–6.

[13] Nielsen JL, Holmgaard S, Jiang N, Englehart KB, Farina D, and Parker PA. Simultaneous and proportional force estimation for multifunction myoelectric prostheses using mirrored bilateral training. IEEE Transactions on Bio-Medical Engineering. 2011;58(3):681–688.

[14] Ison M, Vujaklija I, Whitsell B, Farina D, and Artemiadis P. High-density electromyograph and motor skill learning for robust long-term control of a 7-DoF robot arm. IEEE Transactions on Neural Systems and Rehabilitation Engineering. 2016;24(4):424–433.

[15] Radhakrishnan SM, Baker SN, and Jackson A. Learning a novel myoelectric-controlled interface task. Journal of Neurophysiology. 2008;100(4):2397–2408. PMID: 18667540.

[16] Strazzulla I, Nowak M, Controzzi M, Cipriani C, and Castellini C. Online bimanual manipulation using surface electromyography and incremental learning. IEEE Transactions on Neural Systems and Rehabilitation Engineering. 2017;25(3):227–234.

[17] Hahne JM, Markovic M, and Farina D. User adaptation in myoelectric man-machine interfaces. Scientific Reports. 2017;7(1):4437.

[18] Pistohl T, Cipriani C, Jackson A, and Nazarpour K. Abstract and proportional myoelectric control for multi-fingered hand prostheses. Annals of Biomedical Engineering. 2013;41(12):2687–2698.

[19] Pistohl T, Joshi D, Ganesh G, Jackson A, and Nazarpour K. Artificial proprioceptive feedback for myoelectric control. IEEE Transactions on Neural Systems and Rehabilitation Engineering. 2015;23(3):498–507.

[20] Ghazaei G, Alameer A, Degenaar P, Morgan G, and Nazarpour K. Deep learning-based artificial vision for grasp classification in myoelectric hands. Journal of Neural Engineering. 2017;14(3):036025.

[21] Dyson M, Barnes J, and Nazarpour K. Myoelectric control with abstract decoders. Journal of Neural Engineering. 2018;15(5):056003.

[22] Krasoulis A, Vijayakumar S, and Nazarpour K. Effect of user adaptation on prosthetic finger control with an intuitive myoelectric decoder. Frontiers in Neuroscience. 2019;13:891.

[23] Krasoulis A, Vijayakumar S, and Nazarpour K. Multi-grip classification-based prosthesis control with two EMG-IMU sensors. IEEE Transactions on Neural Systems and Rehabilitation Engineering. 2020;28(2):508–518.

[24] Dyson M, Dupan S, Jones H, and Nazarpour K. Learning, generalisation, scalability of abstract myoelectric control. IEEE Transactions on Neural Systems and Rehabilitation Engineering. 2020;28(7):1539–1547.

[25] Krasoulis A and Nazarpour K. Discrete action control for prosthetic digits. bioRxiv. 2020. Available from: https://www.biorxiv.org/content/early/2020/04/03/2020.03.25.007203.

[26] Hahne JM, Dähne S, Hwang HJ, Müller KR, and Parra LC. Concurrent adaptation of human and machine improves simultaneous and proportional myoelectric control. IEEE Transactions on Neural Systems and Rehabilitation Engineering. 2015;23(4):618–627.

[27] Spanias JA, Perreault EJ, and Hargrove LJ. Detection of and compensation for EMG disturbances for powered lower limb prosthesis control. IEEE Transactions on Neural Systems and Rehabilitation Engineering. 2015;24(2):226–234.

[28] Rahimi A, Benatti S, Kanerva P, Benini L, and Rabaey JM. Hyperdimensional biosignal processing: A case study for EMG-based hand gesture recognition. In: 2016 IEEE International Conference on Rebooting Computing (ICRC). IEEE; 2016. p. 1–8.

[29] Ameri A, Scheme E, Kamavuako E, Englehart K, and Parker P. Real-time, simultaneous myoelectric control using force and position-based training paradigms. IEEE Transactions on Biomedical Engineering. 2014;61(2):279–287.

[30] Fang Y, Zhou D, Li K, and Liu H. Interface prostheses with classifier-feedback-based user training. IEEE Transactions on Biomedical Engineering. 2017;64(11):2575–2583.

[31] Thomas N, Ung G, McGarvey C, and Brown JD. Comparison of vibrotactile and joint-torque feedback in a myoelectric upper-limb prosthesis. Journal of NeuroEngineering and Rehabilitation. 2019;16(1):70.

[32] Guémann M, Bouvier S, Halgand C, *et al.* Sensory and motor parameter estimation for elbow myoelectric control with vibrotactile feedback. Annals of Physical and Rehabilitation Medicine. 2018;61:e467.

[33] Markovic M, Schweisfurth MA, Engels LF, Farina D, and Dosen S. Myocontrol is closed-loop control: Incidental feedback is sufficient for scaling the prosthesis force in routine grasping. Journal of NeuroEngineering and Rehabilitation. 2018;15(1):81.

[34] Oskoei MA and Hu H. Myoelectric control systems – A survey. Biomedical Signal Processing and Control. 2007;2(4):275–294.

[35] Cordella F, Ciancio AL, Sacchetti R, *et al.* Literature review on needs of upper limb prosthesis users. Frontiers in Neuroscience. 2016;10:209. Available from: https://www.frontiersin.org/article/10.3389/fnins.2016.00209.

[36] Sartori M, Durandau G, Došen S, and Farina D. Robust simultaneous myoelectric control of multiple degrees of freedom in wrist-hand prostheses by real-time neuromusculoskeletal modeling. Journal of Neural Engineering. 2018;15(6):066026. Available from: https://doi.org/10.10882F1741-25522Faae26b.

[37] Powell M, Kaliki R, and Thakor N. User training for pattern recognition-based myoelectric prostheses: Improving phantom limb movement consistency and distinguishability. IEEE Transactions on Neural Systems and Rehabilitation Engineering. 2014;22(3):522–532.

[38] Jiang N, Dosen S, Muller K, and Farina D. Myoelectric control of artificial limbs – Is there a need to change focus? IEEE Signal Processing Magazine. 2012;29(5):152–150.

[39] Hwang HJ, Hahne J, and Mueller KR. Real-time robustness evaluation of regression based myoelectric control against arm position change and donning/doffing. PLoS One. 2017;12(11):e0186318.

[40] Vidovic MMC, Hwang HJ, Amsuess S, Hahne JM, Farina D, and Muller KR. Improving the robustness of myoelectric pattern recognition for upper limb prostheses by covariate shift adaptation. IEEE Transactions on Neural Systems and Rehabilitation Engineering. 2016;24(9):961–970.

[41] Zhu X, Liu J, Zhang D, Sheng X, and Jiang N. Cascaded adaptation framework for fast calibration of myoelectric control. IEEE Transactions on Neural Systems and Rehabilitation Engineering. 2017;25(3):254–264.

[42] Hargrove L, Englehart K, and Hudgins B. A training strategy to reduce classification degradation due to electrode displacements in pattern recognition based myoelectric control. Biomedical Signal Processing and Control. 2008;3(2):175–180.

[43] Huang Q, Yang D, Jiang L, et al. A novel unsupervised adaptive learning method for long-term electromyography (EMG) pattern recognition. Sensors. 2017;17(6):1370.

[44] Betthauser JL, Hunt CL, Osborn LE, et al. Limb position tolerant pattern recognition for myoelectric prosthesis control with adaptive sparse representations from extreme learning. IEEE Transactions on Biomedical Engineering. 2018;65(4):770–778.

[45] Amsuess S, Paredes LP, Rudigkeit N, Graimann B, Herrmann MJ, and Farina D. Long term stability of surface EMG pattern classification for prosthetic control. In: 2013 35th Annual International Conference of the IEEE Engineering in Medicine and Biology Society (EMBC); 2013. p. 3622–3625.

[46] Sensinger JW, Lock BA, and Kuiken TA. Adaptive pattern recognition of myoelectric signals: Exploration of conceptual framework and practical algorithms. IEEE Transactions on Neural Systems and Rehabilitation Engineering. 2009;17(3):270–278.

[47] Chen X, Zhang D, and Zhu X. Application of a self-enhancing classification method to electromyography pattern recognition for multifunctional prosthesis control. Journal of NeuroEngineering and Rehabilitation. 2013;10(1):44.

[48] Yeung D, Farina D, and Vujaklija I. Directional forgetting for stable co-adaptation in myoelectric control. Sensors. 2019;19(9):2203. Available from: https://www.mdpi.com/1424-8220/19/9/2203.

[49] Hahne JM, Schweisfurth MA, Koppe M, and Farina D. Simultaneous control of multiple functions of bionic hand prostheses: Performance and robustness in end users. Science Robotics. 2018;3(13):eaat3630.

[50] Ameri A, Akhaee MA, Scheme E, and Englehart K. Regression convolutional neural network for improved simultaneous EMG control. Journal of Neural Engineering. 2019;16(3):036015.

[51] Paaßen B, Schulz A, Hahne J, and Hammer B. Expectation maximization transfer learning and its application for bionic hand prostheses. Neurocomputing. 2018;298:122–133.

[52] Braun DA, Waldert S, Aertsen A, Wolpert DM, and Mehring C. Structure learning in a sensorimotor association task. PLoS One. 2010;5(1):1–8. Available from: https://doi.org/10.1371/journal.pone.0008973.

[53] Nishikawa D, Yu W, Yokoi H, and Kakazu Y. On-line learning method for EMG prosthetic hand control. Electronics and Communications in Japan (Part III: Fundamental Electronic Science). 2001;84(10):35–46. Available from: https://onlinelibrary.wiley.com/doi/abs/10.1002/ecjc.1040.

[54] Müller JS, Vidaurre C, Schreuder M, Meinecke FC, Von Bünau P, and Müller KR. A mathematical model for the two-learners problem. Journal of Neural Engineering. 2017;14(3):036005.

[55] Igual C, Igual J, Hahne JM, and Parra LC. Adaptive auto-regressive proportional myoelectric control. IEEE Transactions on Neural Systems and Rehabilitation Engineering. 2019;27(2):314–322.

[56] Couraud M, Cattaert D, Paclet F, Oudeyer PY, and Rugy Ad. Model and experiments to optimize co-adaptation in a simplified myoelectric control system. Journal of Neural Engineering. 2018;15(2):026006.

Chapter 9

Child prosthetics – a perspective

Matthew Dyson[1], Gemma Wheeler[2], Joe Langley[2],
Abigail Needham[3], Nathaniel Mills[3] and John Head[4]

Research into myoelectric upper limb prosthetics has focussed on algorithmic approaches to decoding muscle signals. A cursory search of PubMed indicates that the ratio of upper limb myoelectric papers focussed on prosthesis control to those which mention children is approximately 20–1. Of those papers which mention children, only a subset focusses on paediatric upper limb prostheses. A similar ratio exists between control algorithms publications and research on myoelectric upper limb sockets. These disparities are likely to reflect the differences in the barriers to entry for various types of research, and the overall time commitments necessary to obtain and validate sufficient data for publication.

The majority of information surrounding myoelectric upper limb prosthetics for children is anecdotal. This reflects the fact that active upper limb prosthetics is a relatively small field, both clinically and academically, of which paediatrics is an even smaller section. As the overall area is small, technical research, whether performed in academia, commercial enterprises, or by non-profits, very rarely reaches or involves the clinical teams necessary to validate developments and evidence efficacy.

This chapter summarises conversations between researchers working in healthcare and academia linked through membership of the Starworks Network, a UK National Institute for Health Research initiative to accelerate the translation of child prosthetics research into daily use. Specifically, it aims to unpack challenges identified by the network and critically analyse the current 'state of the art' in relevant upper limb myoelectric prostheses areas, informed by multiple perspectives. Each section outlines an area of emerging influence over the past decade which is likely to remain influential over the next. It begins with a brief introduction to the Starworks Network and concludes with recommendations from the authors.

[1]School of Engineering, Newcastle University, Newcastle upon Tyne, UK
[2]Lab4Living, Sheffield Hallam University, Sheffield, UK
[3]NIHR Devices for Dignity MedTech Co-operative, Royal Hallamshire Hospital, Sheffield, UK
[4]School of Health and Society, University of Salford, Salford, UK

Starworks

The Starworks Network was established in 2016 as a response to 'market failure' within child prosthetics. Traditional market forces cannot drive innovation in a field characterised by low patient numbers and the highly individualised and rapidly changing needs of children with the result that this group is under-represented in upper limb prosthesis design. In the early stages of the network, the focus was to bring together key stakeholders from across the United Kingdom comprising children and families, academics, healthcare professionals and industry experts to better understand the real, day-to-day challenges of children who use prosthetics. A co-design approach was taken to facilitate reflection and mutual learning between these different stakeholders, as well as early ideation and concept development.

Discussion and activities within the Starworks Network considered live experiences of children, their daily routines and their wider life context, including school, home life, impact on siblings, socialising and hobbies. This was complemented by experiences from healthcare professionals concerning the life course of the child as their growth, and what is needed from the prosthesis technically as well as insights from industry and academia, as to what would be technically possible. This work helped to highlight previously unmet needs as well as gave a more rounded, child-focussed, 'real life' understanding of existing research priorities such as socket fit, adapting to the rapid growth rates of children, personalisation, individualisation, regulation and, crucially, the unique needs of upper limb prosthesis users.

9.1 Co-design

Co-design, or 'the creativity of designers and people not trained in design working together in the design development process' [1], has become somewhat of a buzzword in recent years but in fact has a rich heritage, emerging from the field of participatory design with roots in the civil rights movements of the 1960s and 1970s [2]. As it has moved into more complex contexts such as healthcare and involved a wider range of potentially vulnerable stakeholder groups such as children, the field has matured and demonstrated several strengths that made it particularly relevant to initiatives developing child prosthetics. These include

- principles that give equal value to the contributions of different stakeholders, positioning each as 'virtuosos of their own experience' [3];
- a vast catalogue of tools and methods to create a 'common language' between disparate stakeholder groups, with a focus on flattening hierarchies and addressing potentially stifling power dynamics [4], for example, between children and adults, or between managers and the front-line healthcare staff; and
- skills and activities to elicit hard to reach knowledge, such as tacit, experiential and institutional [5]. This is particularly important with embodied technology such as prosthetics, and complex contexts such as prosthetics services. Considering these different types of knowledge from a range of stakeholders is key to getting to the crux of the problem quicker, to inform the design of new products and technologies, and to anticipate barriers to implementation.

A co-design approach was utilised and promoted throughout the Starworks Network [6]. Limbitless Solutions also employs a modified participatory design approach when creating a prosthesis which they term 'cooperative expression' [7]. While co-design aligns well with rapid pace enterprise-based innovation, achieving similar iterative progress in academia can be challenging. Emergent properties of co-design make the process inherently unpredictable. Although academics and funding bodies will often affirm that the public should play an active role in health research, they usually do so within environments that favour the traditional progression of a lead investigator's pre-existing ideas by promoting detailed project planning and linear progression with fixed milestones.

9.2 Additive manufacturing

The last decade saw an explosion of interest in using additive manufacturing, commonly referred to as 3D printing, to produce upper limb prosthetics for children. Proponents of 3D-printed child prosthetics often cite open-source designs, individualisation and low manufacturing costs as core advantages over traditional methods.

The origins of this approach largely lie in the distributed, open-source community e-NABLE [8]. e-NABLE open-sourced a design for the first 3D-printed child prosthetic in January 2013. In March 2013, Joel Gibbard started the open-source 'Open Hand Project' initiative [9]. Two of the most influential organisations in 3D-printed child prosthetics, Limbitless Solutions [10] and Open Bionics [11], were both founded in 2014. Limbitless Solutions, a non-profit organisation founded by Albert Manero, focusses on child prosthetics. Open Bionics is a private 3D-printed prosthetics company founded by Joel Gibbard and Samantha Payne. The original team at Limbitless Solutions were e-NABLE volunteers, while Open Bionics is the commercial continuation of the Open Hand Project.

9.2.1 Open source

While open-source design enabled widely dispersed individuals in the e-NABLE community to produce highly influential prosthetics, the approach is largely incompatible with existing medical device frameworks. A 2016 review of 3D-printed hand prostheses identified 58 distinct designs, of which the majority were intended for children [12]. These designs are often free and regularly updated; however, they are unregulated and untested and are therefore unlikely to be monitored by healthcare professionals [13].

9.2.2 Cost

The cost advantages of 3D printing prosthetics are difficult to establish. Researchers report low manufacturing costs for small print runs as a central advantage of 3D printing [14]. When production is low scale and parts are highly customisable, it is probable that costs can be reduced significantly relative to traditional techniques [15].

However, in more general cases injection moulding is often cheaper than 3D printing [12]. The majority of 3D designs require significant manual labour, and additional customisation incurs time, the commercial viability of large-scale production is therefore questionable [15]. It is likely that the cost benefits of 3D printing low quantities of customised components will be integrated into existing fabrication pipelines.

9.2.3   Bespoke fitting

Many of the advantages of 3D printing child prosthetics relate to bespoke fitting. Paediatric upper limb prosthetics require regular adjustment because children's residual limbs are still growing. Poor socket comfort is the regular reason for prosthesis rejection [16] and poor fit is increasingly recognised as limiting myoelectric control [17]. Additive manufacturing is highly complementary to scanning and allows bespoke parts to be produced rapidly. Various companies now 3D scan residual limbs. For example, Glaze Prosthetics produces 3D-printed sockets and paediatric prosthetics based on this technology [18]. However, there is little evidence to suggest artisan components such as children's transradial myoelectric sockets can be produced to current standards, particularly without the involvement of specialist clinicians.

9.2.4   Individualisation

Printed prosthesis may be scaled in size and also offer aesthetic individualisation in terms of colour and overall appearance [12], allowing for designs tailored towards children [13]. Limitless Solutions provides an artistic customisation service for children based on participatory design. By involving children in the prosthesis design, the system is intended to increase engagement and promote a greater sense of ownership of the new device [7].

9.2.5   Regulation

Many misconceptions surrounding 3D-printed prosthetics relate to regulatory conformity. The often-reported notion of devices being an 'order of magnitude' cheaper is based on the faulty reasoning that component costs drive prostheses' prices. In reality, price reflects multiple sunk costs, not least of which is securing regulatory conformity, along with prospective costs and enterprise overheads. Similarly, lightweight materials are a moot point without evidence of functionality, durability and safety. Prolonged skin contact also requires materials meet ISO standards for biocompatibility, a non-trivial factor which often appears to be misinterpreted or ignored.

In summary, a disparity exists between public perception of 3D-printed child prosthetics and any available scientific evidence. This may be attributable to the leaps made by international teams of innovators using rapid participatory design methods and publishing their research as internet posts and design files, rather than traditional literature. In parallel, a number of projects have moved to meet the demands of regulating 3D-printed prosthetics and these groups have little incentive to publish the evidence generated.

Public perception of 3D-printed child prosthetics is, like the adult market, largely driven by quotes, adverts and media pieces rather than data. Again, akin to the adult market, media reporting on child prosthetics is typically shallow. Of note, reporters usually appear to be naive to the role 'professional' prosthesis users play in marketing devices and of the increasing involvement of multinational companies in driving positive child prosthetics narratives. Should 3D printing proponents validate that commercial demand exists for low-cost upper limb prosthetics for children, they will also invite competition. However, efficient, automated machining centres and advances in computer-aided design and computer-aided manufacturing mean cheaper, faster and more reliable methods of production that may be used to make the next generation of child-focussed devices.

9.3   Socket fit

The fundamental design of sockets for children with upper limb loss is the same as those built for adults. Fluctuation of residual limb volume is a recognised problem in adult amputees [19,20]. Adults who experience lower-limb loss are physiologically unlikely to remain fit and as a result, the residual limb volume is often unstable. A typical solution is to wear differing numbers of liners depending on the time of day. Adult upper limb amputees, irrespective of the nature of the loss, are usually otherwise physiologically fit. Therefore, the residual limb is, relatively speaking, volume stable.

Limb growth in children is continual and the consequences of this must be mitigated in order for the prosthesis to remain functional. Children at the most common transradial level of congenital limb absence are usually provided with a hybrid self-suspending socket that enables a satisfactory range of motion at the elbow, with some degree of comfort, and effective suspension of the prosthesis. Often, the clinician will allow some growing room within the socket, to mitigate against the need for frequent re-socketing and visits to the clinic. However, this means electrodes in myoelectric devices are often looser immediately following socket delivery, that can affect the levels of control and prosthesis functionality. This is one reason why functionality and comfort [21,22], two properties commonly associated with paediatric prosthesis rejection [16,23,24], are often intrinsically linked.

9.3.1   Digital manufacturing

Digital socket manufacturing, or manufacturing based on a digital work flow, often refers to 3D sockets informed by 3D residual limb scans. As mentioned earlier, this type of technology is already used by a number of enterprises, many of whom work in child prosthetics [18,25]. Digital socket manufacturing is based on the premise that automation can produce sockets more cheaply than current techniques [26]. Relative to traditional casting, digitally scanning residual limbs offers numerous benefits, many of which relieve pressure on the prosthesis user [27]. As socket fitment is an irregular occurrence in adults, and because current casting techniques can be time-consuming and arduous, this technology may be considered particularly salient to child prosthetics.

Digital scanning of residual limbs can be performed using mechanical, optical or electromagnetic methods [28] and upper limb sockets have been successfully produced using computer tomography scans [29], optical scanners [26] and traditional casting followed by optical scanning [30]. A key advantage of digitisation is that patient data can be easily retained, meaning subsequent socket modifications do not require additional cast moulds. It is important to note that digital scanning is not an entirely automatic process. In order to create a comfortable and functional well-fitting socket, practical information about soft tissue areas and bony prominences must be collected, in addition to any areas of skin sensitivity [26]. Anecdotal evidence suggests that early claims that scanning could readily supplant casting have not held true, and that this is widely recognised, both in start-up and commercial funding arenas as well as within academia.

9.3.2   Adaptable sockets

The alternative to multiple low-cost sockets are single sockets which adapt to changes in shape over time. The past decade has seen a number of novel innovations in socket design. These innovations do not target children, rather they are applicable to any user for whom changes in residual limb volume are to be expected.

Many adaptive socket designs derive in some way from compression/release-stabilised (CRS) sockets [31,32]. CRS sockets use longitudinal depressions to compress tissue in the residual limb. Compression displaces tissue which would usually sit between the bone and the socket. The effect of this displacement is a reduction in 'lost motion' between bone and socket movement. Relative to traditional sockets, the CRS design is easy to adapt, because only the longitudinal sections need change.

The general idea of pressure adjustable sockets is to control the pressure at the interface of the residual limb. Two such systems were introduced in 2014. Razak *et al.* developed an air splint socket system for transhumeral users [33] which utilised built-in sensors to allow the wearer to adjust pressure via a microcontroller. A transradial socket based on pressure adjustable chambers and a vacuum pump was developed by Sang *et al.* [34]. The socket introduced a novel design concept whereby compression would be increased during prosthesis use and decreased during rest; aiming to enhance both functionality and comfort simultaneously.

9.3.3   Johns Hopkins University

Recent adaptive upper limb socket research has come from Johns Hopkins University. This team developed the first adaptive socket based on automatic closed-loop feedback from region-specific pressures [35]. The Johns Hopkins socket controls four pneumatically actuated independent air bladders, with embedded textile sensors measuring pressure between the socket and the residual limb and an accelerometer providing information about position. Preliminary experiments demonstrate that by continuously monitoring contact pressure, limb position and operating load, dynamic adjustments can be made to ensure reliable attachment across various activities [36].

9.3.4   Salford University

Research at Salford University proposes a more user-friendly alternative to the standard method of simply inserting myoelectric electrodes into fixed housings within the socket walls. Unlike the standard method, where the electrode contacts are intrinsically tied to the mechanics and fit of the entire socket, the contact pressure and alignment of control electrodes in Salford's design can be adjusted independently [22,37]. The child-focussed version of this system is being developed as part of the Starworks project. This approach would enable prosthetists to continue fitting sockets which accommodate growth and provide an adjustable electrode housing to allow electrode alignment and contact pressure to be tuned over time. The overall goal of this project is to develop a housing which can physically decouple the electrode from the socket, thereby reducing the impact of motion artefacts on myoelectric prosthesis control, and also enabling socket comfort and fit to be enhanced without adversely affecting electrode contact.

9.4   Game-based training

Myoelectric control is not perfect. As a consequence, participants typically have to learn to produce patterns of muscle activity that can be readily distinguished by the myoelectric device [38]. In a rehabilitation context, it is widely recognised that patients usually fail to meet the number of movement repetitions required to induce the adaptation necessary for behavioural improvement. Rehabilitation-relevant muscle activities in the context of game-play offer an alternative motivational and engaging method to increase the number of repetitions performed [39]. Games are promising in this context because they can provide challenging, intensive, task-specific conditions necessary to promote the adaptation of behaviour [40]. As with adaptive upper limb sockets, although game-based systems do not target children per se, their potential application in younger adults is clear. There are currently a number of research groups using game-based training systems for myoelectric control.

9.4.1   University of New Brunswick

Game-based training systems for training of myoelectric upper limb prostheses was pioneered at the University of New Brunswick. In highly prescient research, Lovely *et al.* described many of the concepts and challenges of game-based rehabilitation in the late 1980s [41,42]. In more recent times, the team at New Brunswick have used user-centred design involving patients and prosthesis experts to develop a 2D platform-style game based on low-cost hardware [43] and a virtual reality system for training pattern recognition control of upper limb prostheses [44].

9.4.2   Medical University of Vienna

Researchers led by a team at the Medical University of Vienna developed a game-based rehabilitation protocol that used various muscle contract types to control pre-existing games. The game-based protocol was found to improve muscle separability and fine muscle control while being more enjoyable than standard training [45,46]. Following from this, the Vienna team went on to validate a custom game-based home training system designed around rhythm and music [47].

9.4.3 Limbitless Solutions

Limbitless Solutions has developed game-based rehabilitation solutions designed for children. Unlike many other projects, these games are specifically designed to teach proficiency with Limbitless prostheses. In these conditions, the prosthesis can effectively *be* the game controller, blurring the boundary between prosthesis training and prosthesis use. Game design research from Limbitless stresses the importance of training aligned to real-world use [48,49] and initial tests show enhanced performance with relatively short training sessions [50].

9.4.4 Newcastle University

A game-based system for teaching children prosthesis control in the home is being developed at Newcastle University as part of the Starworks project. The game uses a first person perspective and children control the position of a virtual arm mapped to their residual limb and a virtual prosthesis controlled by muscle activity [51]. The game mechanics involve picking up and manipulating objects in a scene and levels are themed around specific aspects of prosthesis control. The most recent version of the game uses a microcontroller to detect arm movement and muscle activity [52].

9.4.5 University of Groningen

Researchers based at the University of Groningen use a systematic experimental approach to investigate whether skills learned in games actually improve prosthesis use [53–56]. Groningen research suggests that myoelectric control is task-specific, and the nature of training is pivotal to understanding whether abilities learned transfer to prosthesis control [53,54]. Although game-based systems can train people to produce desirable EMG activity, this does not appear to directly translate to significant improvements in prosthesis control [56]. The Groningen group proposes that to improve prosthesis control the coupling of action and perception within a game must match reality, and more abstract forms of training are unlikely to work [55].

Leveraging motivation and engagement is a fundamental of game-based rehabilitation. However, this idea is not trivial to implement and the majority of game-based training systems for upper limb rehabilitation suffer from recognised recurring issues, which have been acknowledged for a long time [42,57]. In addition, recent research suggests that the efficacy of game-based rehabilitation will differ depending on design [48,49,53,54] with simulation of reach and grasp tasks becoming a common proposal [48,49,55]. To achieve traction, these design requirements will have to be addressed along with those of the clinical upper limb rehabilitation community [58].

9.5 Recommendations

The following recommendations arise from the topics raised earlier.

9.5.1 Co-design

The meaningful involvement of users and stakeholders (in this case, children, families and prosthetists, alongside academics and industry) is crucial to understanding the crux and complexity of real-world issues more quickly, as well as to develop comprehensive solutions that encourage uptake – all of which are necessary to positively impact upon this previously under-served area of research [59]. The co-design process enables fast-paced innovation within industry and non-profits. Facilitating the same effectiveness within academia requires adaptation. It is important to note that co-design is rarely linear, and the traditional research paths and project plans used by academics and funding bodies often fail to accommodate this. Co-design can also pose a number of challenges for technical projects, where interdependent components may be developed in parallel. In particular, how to ensure users can make informed and unbiased decisions in otherwise specialist domains can be time-consuming.

9.5.2 Additive manufacturing

There is an academic need for evidence supporting a range of claims made about 3D-printed upper limb prosthetics. Materials must be validated for durability during prosthesis use and for safety in the case of breakages. A need exists to determine whether 3D-printed child prosthetics designs provide sufficient grip strength [15]. Academia should provide more robust critique to ensure that unfounded arguments surrounding printed child prosthetics are moderated in the media. Frequent promises of low-cost access to state-of-the-art technology contribute to public misunderstanding and, in the case of child prosthetics, are sometimes questionable.

9.5.3 Socket fit

It is essential to recognise that socket fit is fundamental to upper limb child prosthetics, particularly for myoelectric devices. As fit is a determinant of both comfort, and functionality it is a key predictor of prosthesis rejection in children [16]. Of the transradial amputees referred for prosthesis treatment in the United Kingdom, when discounting those where cause of limb-loss is unrecorded, the majority are congenital [60]. Despite these statistics, knowledge of why prostheses are rejected [16,24] and data supporting the importance of early intervention [61], relatively little research and development has been focussed on socket design. There is a need to develop sockets that can adapt to a child's growth while ensuring sensor contact for control.

9.5.4 Game-based training

Evidence is required to show that skills developed during game-based training transfer to real-world prosthesis use. It is probable that the nature and degree of skill transfer will relate to game mechanics. Given the limited resources available within prosthetics, future development should focus on game styles confirmed to transfer skills. For bespoke training systems, engagement must be addressed: how to design games such that users will be motivated to play in the medium to long-term. It is unlikely that a single solution can address these challenges for all children. This raises a broader question: how best to enable scaling so that research can move from smaller projects with limited longevity towards more viable solutions.

Acknowledgements

This research is supported by the National Institute of Health Research (NIHR) Devices for Dignity MedTech Co-operative (NIHR D4D). The views expressed are those of the author(s) and not necessarily those of the NHS, the NIHR or of the Department of Health.

References

[1]   Sanders E and Stappers PJ. Convivial Toolbox: Generative Research for the Front End of Design. Amsterdam, The Netherlands: BIS Publishers B.V.; 2012.

[2]   Simonsen J and Robertson T. In: Simonsen J, editor. Routledge International Handbook of Participatory Design. Abingdon-on-Thames, UK: Routledge; 2013.

[3]   Sanders E. Virtuosos of the experience domain. In: Proc. of the 2001 IDSA Education Conference. ISDA; 2001.

[4]   Farr M. Power dynamics and collaborative mechanisms in co-production and co-design processes. Critical Social Policy. 2018;38(4):623–644.

[5]   Langley J, Wolstenholme D, and Cooke J. 'Collective making' as knowledge mobilisation: The contribution of participatory design in the co-creation of knowledge in healthcare. BMC Health Services Research. 2018; 18(585):1–10.

[6]   Wheeler G and Mills N. The Starworks Project: Achievements and next steps. In: Proc. of the International Society of Prosthetics and Orthotists UK MS Annual Scientific Meeting (ISPO). ISPO; 2018.

[7]   Manero A, Smith P, Sparkman J, *et al.* Implementation of 3D printing technology in the field of prosthetics: Past, present, and future. International Journal of Environmental Research and Public Health. 2019;16(9):1641.

[8]   e-NABLE [Website]. e-NABLE; 2020 [cited 2020-03-09]. Available from: https://enablingthefuture.org.

[9]   Open Hand Project [Website]. Open Hand Project; 2020 [cited 2020-03-09]. Available from: http://www.openhandproject.org.

[10]   Limbitless Solutions [Website]. Limbitless Solutions; 2020 [cited 2020-03-09]. Available from: https://limbitless-solutions.org.

[11]   Open Bionics [Website]. Open Bionics; 2020 [cited 2020-03-09]. Available from: https://openbionics.com.

[12] Ten Kate J, Smit G, and Breedveld P. 3D-printed upper limb prostheses: A review. Disability and Rehabilitation: Assistive Technology. 2017;12(3): 300–314.

[13] Tanaka KS and Lightdale-Miric N. Advances in 3D-printed pediatric prostheses for upper extremity differences. Journal of Bone and Joint Surgery. 2016;3(15):1320–1326.

[14] Diment LE, Thompson MS, and Bergmann JH. Three-dimensional printed upper-limb prostheses lack randomised controlled trials: A systematic review. Prosthetics and Orthotics International. 2018;42(1):7–13.

[15] Vujaklija I and Farina D. 3D printed upper limb prosthetics. Expert Review of Medical Devices. 2018;15(7):505–512.

[16] Biddis EA and Chau TT. Upper limb prosthesis use and abandonment: A survey of the last 25 years. Prosthetics and Orthotics International. 2017;31(3): 236–257.

[17] Chadwell A, Kenney L, Thies S, Galpin A, and Head J. The reality of myoelectric prostheses: Understanding what makes these devices difficult for some users to control. Frontiers in Neurorobotics. 2017;10(7). doi:10.3389/fnbot.2016.00007.

[18] Glaze Prosthetics [Website]. Glaze Prosthetics; 2020 [cited 2020-03-09]. Available from: https://glazeprosthetics.com.

[19] Sanders JE, Harrison DS, Allyn KJ, and Myers TR. Clinical utility of in-socket residual limb volume change measurement: Case study results. Prosthetics and Orthotics International. 2009;33(4):378–390.

[20] Sanders JE and Fatone S. Residual limb volume change: Systematic review of measurement and management. Journal of Rehabilitation Research and Development. 2011;48(8):949–986.

[21] Ghoseiri K and Safari MR. Prevalence of heat and perspiration discomfort inside prostheses: Literature review. Journal of Rehabilitation Research and Development. 2014;51(6):855–868.

[22] Head JS, Howard D, Hutchins SW, Kenney L, Heath GH, and Aksenov AY. The use of an adjustable electrode housing unit to compare electrode alignment and contact variation with myoelectric prosthesis functionality: A pilot study. Prosthetics and Orthotics International. 2016;40(1):123–128.

[23] Scotland TR and Galway HR. A long-term review of children with congenital and acquired upper limb deficiency. The Journal of Bone and Joint Surgery British Volume. 1983;65(3):346–349.

[24] Postema K, van der Donk V, van Limbeek J, Rijken RA, and Poelma MJ. Prosthesis rejection in children with a unilateral congenital arm defect. Clinical Rehabilitation. 1999;13(3):243–249.

[25] Ambionics [Website]. Ambionics; 2020 [cited 2020-03-09]. Available from: https://www.ambionics.co.uk.

[26] Strömshed E. The Perfect Fit Development process for the use of 3D technology in the manufacturing of custom-made prosthetic arm sockets [Masters Thesis]. Faculty of Engineering, Lund University. Lund, Sweden; 2016.

[27]   Kratky V. Photogrammetric digital modeling of limbs in orthopaedics. In: Proc. of the ASP Fall Convention. Springer; 1974.

[28]   Sanders JE, Mitchell SB, Zachariah SG, and Wu K. A digitizer with exceptional accuracy for use in prosthetics research: A technical note. Journal of Rehabilitation Research and Development. 2003;40(2):191–195.

[29]   Cabibihan J, Abubasha MK, and Thakor N. A method for 3-D printing patient-specific prosthetic arms with high accuracy shape and size. IEEE Access. 2018;6:25029–25039.

[30]   da Silva LA, Medola FO, Rodrigues OV, Rodrigues ACT, and Sandnes FE. Interdisciplinary-based development of user-friendly customized 3D printed upper limb prosthesis. In: Proc. of the AHFE 2018 International Conferences on Usability & User Experience and Human Factors and Assistive Technology. Springer; 2018.

[31]   Alley RD, Williams 3rd TW, Albuquerque MJ, and Altobelli DE. Prosthetic sockets stabilized by alternating areas of tissue compression and release. Journal of Rehabilitation Research and Development. 2011;48(6): 679–696.

[32]   Alley RD. Adaptable Socket System, Method, and Kit; U.S. Patent 9 283 093 B2, March 15th, 2016.

[33]   Razak NA, Osman NA, Gholizadeh H, and Ali S. Prosthetics socket that incorporates an air splint system focusing on dynamic interface pressure. Biomedical Engineering Online. 2014;13. doi:10.1186/1475-925X-13-108.

[34]   Sang Y, Li X, Gan Y, Su D, and Luo Y. A novel socket design for upper-limb prosthesis. International Journal of Applied Electromagnetics and Mechanics. 2014;45(1–4):881–886.

[35]   Candrea D, Sharma A, Osborn L, Gu Y, and Thakor N. An adaptable prosthetic socket: Regulating independent air bladders through closed-loop control. In: Proc. of the IEEE International Symposium on Circuits and Systems (ISCAS). IEEE; 2017. p. 1–4.

[36]   Gu Y, Yang D, Osborn L, Candrea D, Liu H, and Thakor N. An adaptive socket with auto-adjusting air bladders for interfacing transhumeral prosthesis: A pilot study. Proceedings of the Institution of Mechanical Engineers Part H—Journal of Engineering in Medicine. 2019;233(8):812–822.

[37]   Head J. The effect of socket movement and electrode contact on myoelectric prosthesis control during daily living activities [PhD Thesis]. University of Salford. Salford, UK; 2014.

[38]   Tabor A, Bateman S, Scheme EJ, Flatla DR, and Gerling K. Designing game-based myoelectric prosthesis training. In: CHI '17: Proceedings of the 2017 CHI Conference on Human Factors in Computing Systems. Association for Computing Machinery; 2017.

[39]   Lohse K, Shirzad N, Verster A, Hodges N, and Van der Loos RF. Video games and rehabilitation: Using design principles to enhance engagement in physical therapy. The Journal of Neurologic Physical Therapy. 2013;37(4): 166–175.

[40]   Saposnik G and Levin M. Virtual reality in stroke rehabilitation: A meta-analysis and implications for clinicians. Stroke. 2011;42(5):1380–1386.

[41] Lovely DF, Hruczkowski T, and Scott RN. Computer aided myoelectric training. In: Proceedings of the Engineering in Medicine and Biology Society. IEEE; 1988.

[42] Lovely DF, Stocker D, and Scott RN. A computer-aided myoelectric training system for young upper limb amputees. Journal of Microcomputer Applications. 1990;13(3):245–259.

[43] Tabor A, Bateman S, and Scheme EJ. Game-based myoelectric training. In: CHI PLAY Companion 16: Proceedings of the 2016 Annual Symposium on Computer-Human Interaction in Play Companion Extended Abstracts. Association for Computing Machinery; 2016.

[44] Woodward RB and Hargrove LJ. Adapting myoelectric control in real-time using a virtual environment. Journal of NeuroEngineering and Rehabilitation. 2019;16(11). doi:10.1186/s12984-019-0480-5.

[45] Prahm C, Vujaklija I, Kayali F, Purgathofer P, and Aszmann OC. Game-based rehabilitation for myoelectric prosthesis control. JMIR Serious Games. 2017;5(1):e3.

[46] Prahm C, Kayali F, Vujaklija I, Sturma A, and Aszmann O. Increasing motivation, effort and performance through game-based rehabilitation for upper limb myoelectric prosthesis control. In: Proceedings of the IEEE International Conference on Virtual Rehabilitation (ICVR). IEEE; 2017.

[47] Prahm C, Kayali F, and Aszmann O. MyoBeatz: Using music and rhythm to improve prosthetic control in a mobile game for health. In: Proceedings of the IEEE International Conference on Serious Games and Applications for Health (SeGAH). IEEE; 2019.

[48] Dombrowski M, Smith PA, and Buyssens R. Utilizing digital game environments for training prosthetic use. In: Proceedings of the 8th International Virtual, Augmented and Mixed Reality Conference. Springer; 2016.

[49] Dombrowski M, Smith PA, and Buyssens R. Designing Alternative Interactive Techniques to Aid in Prosthetic Rehabilitation for Children. In: Chung W and Shin CS, editors. Advances in Affective and Pleasurable Design. Advances in Intelligent Systems and Computing. Cham: Springer; 2017.

[50] Manero A, Smith P, Sparkman J, *et al.* Utilizing additive manufacturing and gamified virtual simulation in the design of neuroprosthetics to improve pediatric outcomes. MRS Communications. 2019;9:941–947.

[51] Dyson M and Nazarpour K. Home-based myoelectric training using biofeedback gaming. In: Proc. of the Trent International Prosthetics Symposium (TIPS). ISPO; 2019.

[52] Dyson M, Olsen J, and Nazarpour K. A home-based myoelectric training system for children. In: Proc. of the 20th Myoelectric Controls Symposium (MEC). University of New Brunswick; 2020.

[53] van Dijk L, van der Sluis CK, van Dijk HW, and Bongers RM. Task-oriented gaming for transfer to prosthesis use. IEEE Transactions on Neural Systems and Rehabilitation Engineering. 2016;24(12):1384–1394.

[54] van Dijk L, van der Sluis CK, van Dijk HW, and Bongers RM. Learning an EMG controlled game: Task-specific adaptations and transfer. PLoS One. 2016;11(8):e0160817.

[55]   Heerschop A, van der Sluis CK, Otten E, and Bongers RM. Performance among different types of myocontrolled tasks is not related. Human Movement Science. 2020;3:102592.

[56]   Kristoffersen MB, Franzke AW, van der Sluis CK, Murgia A, and Bongers RM. Serious gaming to generate separated and consistent EMG patterns in pattern recognition prosthesis control. Biomedical Signal Processing and Control; 2020;62. doi:10.1016/j.bspc.2020.102140.

[57]   Flores E, Tobon G, Cavallaro E, Cavallaro FI, Perry JC, and Keller T. Improving patient motivation in game development for motor deficit rehabilitation. In: ACE '08: Proceedings of the 2008 International Conference on Advances in Computer Entertainment Technology. Association for Computing Machinery; 2008.

[58]   Tatla SK, Shirzad N, Lohse KR, *et al.* Therapists' perceptions of social media and video game technologies in upper limb rehabilitation. JMIR Serious Games. 2015;3(1):e2.

[59]   Jones H, Supan S, and Nazarpour K. The future of prosthetics: A user perspective. In: Trent International Prosthetics Symposium. Salford, UK; 2019.

[60]   Limbless Statistics (formerly National Amputee Statistical Database [NAS-DAB] Annual Report 2010–2011) [Website]. United National Institute for Prosthetics and Orthotics Development (UNIPOD); 2013 [cited 2020-03-09]. Available from: http://www.limbless-statistics.org.

[61]   Davids JR, Wagner LV, Meyer LC, and Blackhurst DW. Prosthetic management of children with unilateral congenital below-elbow deficiency. The Journal of Bone and Joint Surgery American Volume. 2006;88(6):1294–1300.

Chapter 10

Design and development of transradial upper limb prosthesis for children with soft-grippers

Daniel De Barrie[1] and Khaled Goher[1]

Upper limb reduction defects occur congenitally in 4.1–5 per 10,000 births [1]. Factoring in non-congenital amputations is problematic, though one long-term study showed dysvascular, trauma-related, and cancer-related conditions had a respective frequency of 2.25, 2.65, and 0.15 per 100,000 between the ages of 0 and 14 years [2]. Despite these figures, active prosthetic devices are routinely only given to adults, with the assumption that myoelectric devices (those controlled by electrical signals generated in the muscles) are difficult to scale down, as well as being too expensive, especially with the frequent replacement schedule that a growing child necessitates [3].

In cases where young children with upper limb amputation utilize a prosthetic device, the child will often develop their own methods of grasping objects [4]. This causes later difficulty adapting to methods using a prosthetic device as the child's motor neural skills and proprioception will have only developed up to the base of the stump. This adaptive grasping can also cause physiological issues in the long term, such as asymmetric posture and muscular–skeletal pain [5] due to an overreliance on the residual limb and off balance centre of mass [6]. Despite the benefits of prosthetic use, rejection remains a major issue. Early fitting has been shown to reduce this risk [7], with one study showing a rejection rate for fitting before and after the age of 2 years of 22% and 58%, respectively [8]. If the usefulness of the device is demonstrated to the child, the rejection rate is greatly reduced; a functional myoelectric device should therefore aid in reducing rejection rates.

The cost of an active prosthetic in high-income nations, such as the United States, is upwards of $20,000 [9], with even simple cosmetic options costing around $3,000–$5,000. In low-income nations, an expense on this scale for a custom fit prosthetic device is totally unfeasible, especially with many families already facing hardship as a result of the amputation [10]. The use of additive manufacturing introduces the prospect of rapidly producing low-cost custom prosthetic devices, such as the ReHand [11] with a production cost below $1,250; this cost may be reduced further should 3D printing be used in conjunction with injection moulding for standardized parts [12]. The technology has already been proven as means of producing myoelectric

[1]BioRobotics and Medical Technologies Laboratory, School of Engineering, University of Lincoln, Lincoln, UK

prosthetics [12], though thus far the paediatric devices have predominantly been open-source body-powered devices, with very limited functionality.

This work presents a myoelectric device for toddlers that can be produced at a low cost while maintaining high grasp performance levels. To achieve this, cable-driven soft-grippers have been integrated into the design, with the intention of improving the grasp contact surface. The soft-grippers also aim to provide a more even distribution of the grasp force, mimicking the grip force distribution of a human hand [13]. The device has been named SIMPA: Soft-grasp Infant Myoelectric Prosthetic Arm.

10.1   Prosthetic design and realization

The design ethos of the project was adapted to prove advanced manufacturing techniques, such as 3D printing, to realize a low-cost yet highly function active prosthetic device. From the outset, the arm was designed, wherever possible, to be directly 3D printed, only utilizing other techniques or external source components where necessary. The design first focused on the development of the grippers, then continued to the hand, forearm, and eventually the socket.

10.1.1   Gripper design

The topic of soft-robotics is an up and coming research topic that has typically focused on the agricultural applications. As the name suggests, this area covers robotic actuators and grippers that perform tasks by deforming their structure. The end effector of this device aims to highlight how soft-grippers can be incorporated into a prosthetic device.

There are numerous styles of soft-grippers, including pneumatic and shape memory materials; in this instance, a cable-driven design was used due to the simplicity of the design and its ability to be incorporated into a small-scale paediatric device.

The gripper design is loosely based on human fingers. The sizing of the gripper is based on the measurements of a 4-year-old child's hand. The extruding section of each finger is 50-mm long and comprises three segments. The base extends a further 20 mm, though this is purely to house the gripper within the hand. The gripper contains within it hollow tubes that allow for a wire or string to be threaded through. When the string is pulled back, the gripper will contract around the slots in the gripper. The total angular deformation of the tip is approximately 180 degrees, due to the two 90-degree slots. Due to the nature of the flexible gripper, the exact deformation is difficult to fully quantify or model. Some lateral deformation is possible with this gripper in cases where an obstruction occurs.

It was decided that the grippers would be constructed as a composite. The gripper is 20-mm wide and is effectively spit in half (Figure 10.1). It features a malleable contact surface and a stiffer silicon rubber that acts as a reinforcement for the gripper, as well as an elastic energy store. For the contact area of the grippers, a malleable material, with a feel resembling that of human skin, is to be used. The justification for this is that the surface of the gripper would distort around an object's surface during a grasp, thus increasing the contact surface area. The material chosen for the

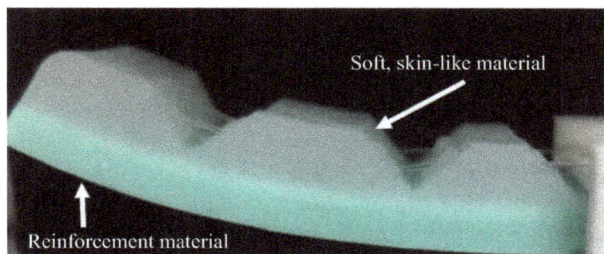

Figure 10.1   Soft-gripper design with composite structure highlighted

contact surface was Dragon Skin™ 30 (Smooth-On, Inc.). This silicon rubber is used in prosthetic makeup for its skin-like appearance and texture; this skin-like property should be well suited for this application.

The second component of the composite gripper is Smooth-Sil™ 960 (Smooth-On, Inc.). This material acts as an elastic energy store for returning the gripper back to its pre-deformation state. Smooth-Sil 960 is a more rigid silicon rubber than the Dragon Skin 30 and is not intended to come into contact with objects during a grasp. The material also acts as a reinforcement for the gripper, with the base extension also being made from this material so that the gripper may be securely slotted into the 'hand' of the prosthetic.

Unlike the rest of the device, the grippers were not 3D printed directly and were instead moulded. An inverse CAD model was used for the mould, which was then 3D printed. The production of these grippers is a straightforward process that has been able to achieve consistent results.

A variant of the gripper was also produced using the same CAD, 3D printing and moulding process. This version has two segments, rather than three, mimicking the style of a thumb. The main reasoning behind, including this variant gripper, was to improve the biomimicry of the hand to make the device more cosmetically appealing. This gripper would only be used as a thumb with the remaining digits acting as fingers with three segments.

10.1.2   Forearm and hand

Due to the limitations in the moulding of the grippers, a three-digit hand is required. This hand is composed of three slots for the grippers, two for the fingers and one for the thumb. These are offset from each over by 90 degrees. Within the hand, there are channels that allow the cable to be threaded through the hand into the forearm of the device. The back of the hand has an open slot which allows access in order for the cables to be attached to the actuators.

The forearm houses two Actuonix PQ12 Micro Linear Actuator (Actuonix Motion Devices Inc.). A single actuator is dedicated to thumb actuation, with the other reserved for the fingers. The 1:63 gear ratio version was chosen for this application. This provides a maximum output of 30 N with a stroke speed of 8 mm/s. The forearm also houses the rest of the electronic components. This comprises primarily a 7.5 V 2.2 A h battery, an Arduino Nano, and an OYMotion Gravity: Analog EMG Sensor (OYMotion Technologies, Inc.). The OYMotion Gravity is an armband-based surface electromyography (sEMG). The device rests on the user's bicep and records the muscular activity in order to control the device.

The forearm and forearm cover both have been designed with slots to accommodate the components. This allows for easy installation and replacement of parts, in keeping with the desire to produce a modular device. The arm is also designed held together with nylon bolts in this initial prototype device, allowing for rapid assembly/disassembly.

10.1.2.1 Socket design

The traditional method of preforming this involves using a plaster cast of the residual limb. The process aims to capture the dimensional data of the stump, so that the produced socket fits exactly; failure to do so will result discomfort and slippage, rendering prosthetic unusable. Various studies have shown that comfort ranks among one of the most important factors when rating the performance of a prosthetic device [14]. The casting process relies heavily on the skill of the prosthetist and on the stump being kept stationary during casing. In the case of young children, this lengthy casing process is often traumatic and uncomfortable; this, in turn, affects the quality of the cast, as the child is likely to move around during the lengthy procedure. The high growth rate too proves problematic as by the time the stump has been produced, the child may have outgrown it. This project proposes an alternative that utilizes 3D scanning and CAD modelling to design and manufacture the socket without the need for the lengthy casting process.

To prototype the SIMPA socket, a scan was taken off the residual limb of a 4-year-old boy who had undergone transradial below-elbow amputation. The socket (Figure 10.2) was modelled based on this scan, utilizing the *Mesh* feature within Autodesk Fusion 360 (Autodesk, Inc.). The inner socket was designed to closely match the stump geometry, with a widened opening at the top to allow the socket to be fitted to the stump. The socket, along with the rest of the arm, is manufactured from acrylonitrile butadiene styrene (ABS) for this initial prototype device.

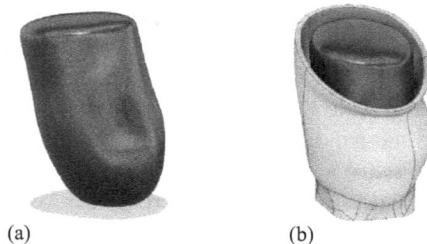

(a)   (b)

Figure 10.2   3D scan of residual limb (a), CAD rendering of the socket (b)

Moving forward the internal layer would be printed from a softer material, such as thermoplastic polyurethane.

10.1.2.2   3D printing

The final socket design was incorporated with the previously designed arm into a single CAD model (Figure 10.3). This model was then printed as one complete unit comprising the socket, forearm, and hand. The print time, with an infill of 25%, a layer height of 0.1 mm, and a support structure, was approximately 40 h. The part was oriented such that the layers follow the direction of the forearm. This is to provide maximum strength in the load-supporting direction. Unlike injection moulding with its uniform structure, design for additive manufacturing must consider this layer direction factor.

The other components, the forearm cover and hand backplate, were printed separately to the main body of the device. The backplate includes 3D-printed detailing, with the name of the device, SIMPA, embossed in blue ABS. The use of dual extrusion allows for this kind of appearance customization, without the need for additional processing. All the parts printed with a high-quality finish and with the only finishing technique required being the removal of the support structures.

10.1.3   Control system

A voluntary opening control system has been integrated with the prosthetic. This system utilizes a single EMG sensor site on the upper arm. The system is Arduino-based and programmed via Simulink® (The MathWorks, Inc.).

The basic outline of the circuit design (Figure 10.4) centres on an Arduino board acting as the controller. The primary input into the device comes in the form of an OYMotion Gravity sEMG sensor. This input will be processed by the controller, so that a recorded muscle flexion sends a positive signal to the actuators, causing the grasp to open. The inverse is true when no flexion is recorded, with the grasp closing. The second input to the controller is from the linear actuators built in potentiometers. These provide a resistance value that correlates to the shaft position; this allows for grasp open and closed limits to be set, as well as the incorporation of a rudimentary grasp detection system.

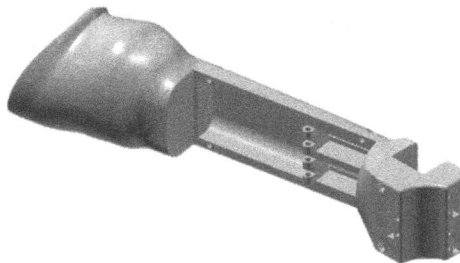

Figure 10.3   CAD model of the combined socket, forearm, and hand

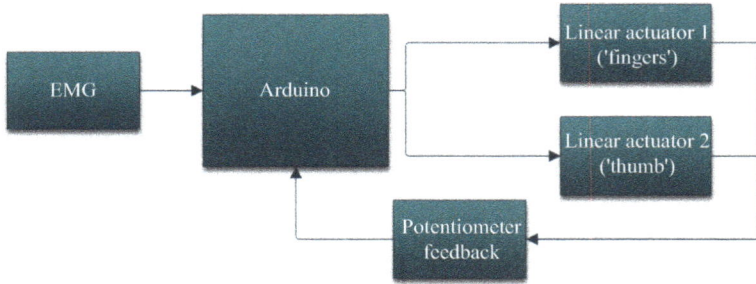

Figure 10.4 Block diagram outlining the control system

10.1.3.1 Grasp detection

A grasp detection system has been implemented to determine if an obstruction has occurred that has caused the actuator to slow to a near stall. This is to prevent the motor from burning out when an object is grasped, as ordinarily the actuator would continue to be driven in an attempt to retract until the limit is reached.

The built-in potentiometer detects the position of the shaft: if the difference from a previous reading is considered, then the speed and direction of the shaft extension can be determined. The system utilizes this so that when an obstruction, i.e. a grasp, occurs and the speed of the shaft is slowed below a set value, the system shuts off the power to the motors to hold them in their current position. Figure 10.5 shows the speed of the shaft (bottom) and the binary output for this subsystem (top). The system can be adjusted so that even a slight obstruction causes the motors to stall. In its current set-up, the threshold is 2.9 mm/s or 19% of the actuator's published maximum shaft travel speed. In this configuration, objects such as a soft toy will be detected as a grasp once the object has experienced a small amount of deformation.

10.1.3.2 Surface electromyography

EMG is the process of recording electrical signals produced by muscles under flexion. The technique has been widely adopted in medical applications [15], including prosthetic control. The present system uses surface EMG, where electrodes on the surface of the skin record the voltage difference created by muscle activity.

The sEMG can be broken down further into four subcategories:

- Single-site, single-action: this system uses a single detection site which preforms an action once a single threshold is met, e.g. opening a grasp.
- Single-site, multi-action: this is the same as the previous system; however, here the amplitude of the signal is taken into account, e.g. different grasps for low-level, mid-level, and high-level signals.
- Multi-site, single-action: here multiple sEMG sites are used to create a more robust detection system; only a single action would be performed with this method.

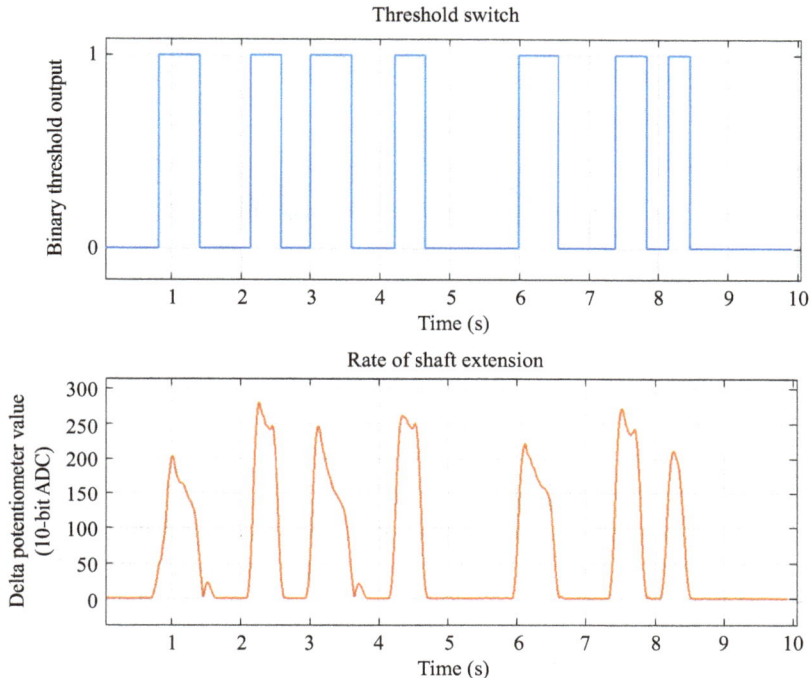

Figure 10.5　Speed of actuator shaft extension (bottom), grasp threshold switch output (top)

- Multi-action, multi-site: this is the most advanced method of sEMG whereby multiple sites are used, each with a different action, e.g. different grasp types, wrist or elbow actuation, etc.

The OYMotion Gravity was used to record the sEMG signals. The sensor was placed approximately on the centre of the bicep. The sEMG location is due to this prototype design being based around a high-level transradial amputee, with an insufficiently sized residual limb for forearm-based recording. A 23-year-old male of average build was used during the development and initial testing of the system in order to prove the concept. Future validation with an age-appropriate subject is planned. Raw data was collected of the muscle flexing and relaxing over a period of approximately 10 s, as shown in Figure 10.6.

The raw recording averages around 300 on the Arduino's analogue input scale (10-bit ADC, 0–1,023). The raw data was first normalized around 0 and set to an absolute scale, so that the activity is contained within the positive region. This normalized data still contained a large amount of noise. A moving average filter was incorporated here to smoothen the data.

The final step in the processing of the sEMG recording was to incorporate an Interval Test Block. This determines if the average value over a given amount of time

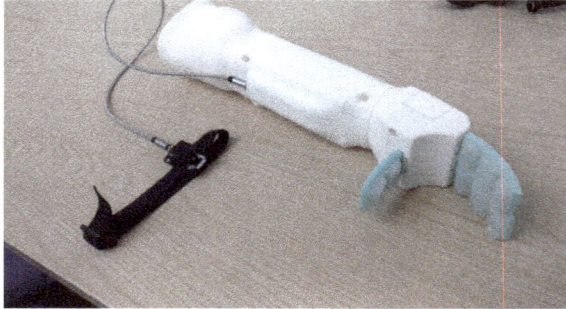

Figure 10.6   The assembled SIMPA working prototype

is within set boundaries, producing a binary output. This boundary condition would be adjusted per the individual's recorded muscular activity. In instances where a child is first exposed to the system, a low sensitivity value might aid in initially presenting the function of the device, with the sensitivity later being reduced as the user familiarizes themselves with the system and its required muscle flexion/relaxation.

When the sEMG system outputs a HIGH signal, the hand begins to open and this will continue until the set maximum limit of the actuator is met. For the fingers, the actuator traverses between 0 mm extension for fully closed and 19 mm for fully open. The thumb, meanwhile, has limits of 5–19 mm for closed and open, respectively. This open–close hand transition takes approximately 2.3 s, with closed to open averaging 2.1 s.

The final Simulink model provides a control system that can easily be adjusted to meet the users' specific requirements based on their sEMG data. Grasp limits and thresholds are also easily reprogrammable and should design changes to the grippers take place.

10.1.3.3   Final assembly

The design of the arm is intentionally modular. This allows for the components, including the internal electrical parts, to simply slot into place. The cables are threaded through the grippers and tied to the end of linear actuators' shaft. The sEMG chip is slotted into the forearm cover and is connected to the rest of the circuit. Finally, nylon nut and bolts are used to secure the covers to the main structure, resulting in the working prototype shown in Figure 10.6.

The advantage of the modular design is 2-fold: first, it allows for the easy replacement of components should they fail; second, it allows for some of the parts to move across when the child has outgrown their current device and requires a new slightly larger device utilizing the same internal components.

The final device has the battery capacity of continuously running the actuators and other electric components for 6.6 h, with a standby time of 33 h. Currently, the battery must be removed to charge, though this would be revised in future versions of the device.

10.1.4 Experimental procedure

For the experimental procedures, the device was controlled via a button-based system to allow for easier operation; the rest of the device remains consistent with the previously detailed design. Due to restrictions, the device has not been directly verified by its target audience; however, the procedure detailed here covers the initial verification for the use of soft-grippers in a paediatric prosthetic device.

The experimental procedure for the device covered the grasping of objects with various geometry, with the success and failure noted. The arm also performed some examples of activities of daily living (ADL). To determine the approximate grasping force of the hand, three methods have been employed. The first uses weighted objects. The second measures the pinch force directly, and the third utilizes the Takei Physical Fitness Test: Grip-A (Takei Scientific Instruments Co., Ltd).

10.1.4.1 Object grasp test

In this experimental procedure, a number of objects were grasped using the prosthetic (Figure 10.7). These objects vary in size, shape, and weight, comprising geometric shapes and everyday objects. The test procedure was to grasp each object ten times. The orientation of the grasp is varied and the successfulness of each is noted. The objects are in almost all cases grasped directly from the workbench, in the case of the pen and wooden stick, some manual orientation is performed prior to a grasp. Once grasped, the arm is steadily shaken for a period of 10 s, this is to replicate the movement of the user while holding an object. If after this 10-s period had elapsed, the object is still securely held within the hand, then the grasp is deemed to be successful.

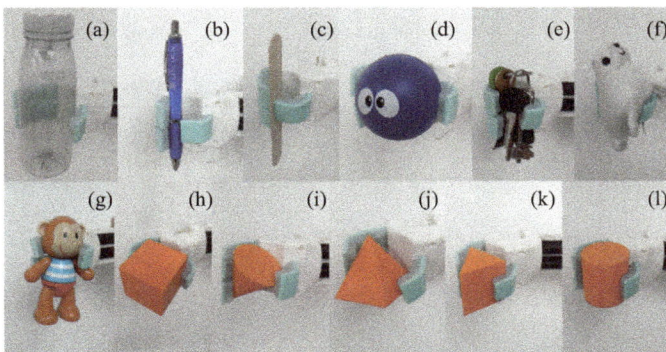

Figure 10.7   SIMPA grasping tasks: plastic bottle (a), pen (b), wooden stick (c), sponge ball (d), set of keys (e), soft toy (f), hard plastic toy (g), cube (h), cone (i), pyramid (j), triangular prism (k) and cylinder (l)

The experiment is performed with both the two-segment and the three-segment thumb set-ups; the results for both are noted in Table 10.1.

10.1.4.2   Activities of daily living

These procedures do not provide numerical results and mostly act as a demonstration for how the device may be incorporated into the daily life of the user. The tasks were performed with both two-segment and three-segment thumb gripper configurations, though as there was no notable difference between the performances of the two, only the two-segment referenced in the results.

Writing task was performed, this required a secure and stable grasp of the pen. With correct positioning the device is able to do this, with the pen secured strongly enough to apply the pressure required to mark the paper.

This next task required a bottle to be grasped using a standard cylindrical grip. The bottle is then tilled over a container and the water is poured in. The test requires the hand to have a secure grip of the bottle, especially as the mass and centre of gravity shift during the pour. The prosthetic arm in both gripper configurations is able to grasp the bottle and pour the liquid without any issues. This performance is likely indicative of the device's ability to perform other ADLs such as drinking from a vessel.

This final procedure shows the prosthetics ability to accurately place objects. Across all of the objects and gripper configurations, the arm is able to perform the task with ease. The device is able to grasp from multiple angles and as such the grasp can be positioned in such a way as to place the objects in their appropriate slot. The procedure highlights how the device might be used in everyday grasping tasks.

Table 10.1   Result of object grasp test

Test item	Object mass (g)	Grasp success rate (%)	
		Three segments	Two segments
Plastic water bottle (empty)	20.6	100	100
Plastic water bottle (250 ml)	270.6	100	100
Pen	11.5	100	100
Wooden stick	2.7	60	60
Sponge ball	23.7	100	100
Set of keys	94.2	80	50
Soft toy	21.3	100	90
Hard plastic toy	56	90	80
Cube	31	100	100
Cone	9	60	50
Pyramid	13.2	60	60
Tri-prism	13.2	80	80
Cylinder	20.4	100	100
Average		87	82

10.1.4.3 Weighted object test

This procedure used 3D-printed objects with weights attached to them to determine the lifting capacity of the device. Four 3D-printed objects featuring loops on which to hook weights on were used. The point at which slippage occurs when the device is stationary is presented in Table 10.2.

10.1.4.4 Pinch force test

This experiment was set-up to determine the pinch force of the grippers. The intention is to compare with published results of both biological grasping force and other prosthetic hands. The test utilized a set of high accuracy scales, perched on a stand, which can be pinched by the grippers. The pinch test is performed by closing the grasp of the prosthetic, thus applying a force that can be read on the scale. The test is performed under three system configurations:

- Actuators-on: under this configuration, the motor is continuously powered during the grasp;
- Actuators-off: in this instance, the grasp is performed and then the actuators are powered down before its reading is taken;
- Grasp detection system active: here the grasp detection system is active, automatically powering down the actuators once a grasp has been recorded.

The procedure was repeated ten times for each configuration, with an average result being calculated from these readings, as presented in Table 10.3.

10.1.5 Grip strength test

The grasp force of the device was determined using the Takei Physical Fitness Test: Grip-A. The system uses an analogue dial to display the grasp force. The force is applied by pulling the bar connected to the dial towards the base of the frame. This bar is adjustable in order to meet a range of hand sizes. The grasp test is conduced ordinarily by having the user apply their full strength, with the dial indicating the maximum force recorded. In the case of the prosthetic, the same procedure is used, with handle being adjusted to fit the device. The test was performed with both the grasp detection active and disabled with the results displayed in Table 10.4.

Table 10.2 Result of weighted object test

Object		Two-segment thumb (N)	Three-segment thumb (N)
44 m	Cylinder	5.36	5.36
22.5 m	Cylinder	5.7	3.7
Triangular	Prism	9.77	5.77
Pinch grasp		2.76	2.3
Average		5.9	4.3

Table 10.3   Results of pinch force test

Run	Motor (powered)	Motor (unpowered)	Grip detection
1	8.63	5.84	3.82
2	8.78	5.64	3.73
3	8.88	5.89	3.94
4	8.49	5.45	3.78
5	8.42	5.49	3.85
6	8.56	5.74	3.93
7	8.29	5.25	3.87
8	8.39	5.40	3.92
9	8.26	5.15	3.76
10	8.63	5.59	3.96
Average	8.5	5.5	3.9

Table 10.4   Results of the grasp strength test: grip detection system (GDS)

Run	GDS disabled (N)	GDS active (N)
1	4.91	1.96
2	4.91	1.96
3	4.91	2.94
4	4.91	2.94
5	4.91	1.96
6	4.91	2.94
7	4.91	1.96
8	4.91	2.94
9	4.91	1.96
10	4.91	1.96
Average	4.91	2.35

10.1.6   Conclusions and further work

The present device is developed specifically with the intention of showcasing the viability of an active prosthetic device suitable for young children. The device is thought to be the first myoelectric prosthetic arm for children under 5 to be 3D printed. It is also first prosthetic arm to incorporate soft-grippers, even when adult devices are explored.

A key reason for the use of 3D printing in the project is to reduce the cost and lead-times associated with prosthetic devices. This is implemented out of a desire to encourage healthcare providers such as the NHS, to consider the adoption of a policy based around early prosthetic fitting in order to reduce rejection rates. Currently cost ranks among the top reasons for active prosthetics are not being fitted at as soon as the child has developed enough to use such a device. The material cost of producing the device was around £500, including scrappage and prototypes. This represents a significant reduction in cost compared to the current production myoelectric devices, though it is worth noting that the overheads have not been considered in this instance. The final cost on the device would vary slightly depending on the specific config-uration based around the end user and the production scalability of standard parts, such as the grippers. There may also be a labour cost reduction thanks to the speed at which 3D-scan-based socket modelling can be performed and the predominantly automated process of 3D printing.

The other major reason is the often poor performance of paediatric devices. With the primary focus, even within scientific literature being on adult devices, their paediatric and in particular toddler-sized counterparts are often neglected, with no significant improvements in design over the last few decades. Adult and adolescent scale devices have started to make use of advanced technologies such as 3D printing to improve on past designs. Similarly, the topic of robotics has developed greatly in a number of ways. With regards to this project, the adoption of cheap, small-scale control units such as Arduino boards and the upcoming field of soft robotics are of particular interest. The present design takes the concept of 3D-printing myoelec-tric devices, using Arduino-based control and soft-grippers, to produce a prosthetic that is highly capable while remaining low cost, highly customizable, and easy to manufacture device.

The results from the experimental procedures presented provide early validation that this novel approach to prosthetic design is plausible and may be advantageous, particularly in the case of small-scale paediatric devices. The use of soft-grippers as a prosthetic end device is thought to be unexplored within current literature. The use of the grippers in this device was intended to allow for a flexible grasp, which also utilizes a malleable contact surface. To this end, the grippers have worked as desired. Looking at the results of the grasp tests, it is observed that the grippers can grasp all of the objects available. On some of the objects, such as the plastic toy, the grippers can be seen to deform around the object, increasing the contact area and thus improving the grasp. An additional value to the use of the grippers is the safety factor. In more tradition grippers, joints would be used to facilitate the movement. These joints can create pinch points, which would present a hazard to the user, particularly as the target audience is young children. The soft-grippers remove the risk posited by pinch points. The grasp detection mechanism along with the soft material of the grippers, also reduces the risk of injury should the user grasp a part of their own body or another individual.

One limitation of the grasp effectiveness is the maximum force produced by the micro-linear actuators. The maximum force recorded during the pinch test was 8.5 N with the motor continuously powered. Comparing this to each motors' maximum-rated output of 30 N demonstrates the losses within the system required to deform the grippers. The contact area deformation too is thought to hinder the application of the force, as some of the energy will be stored as elastic potential, rather than directly acting on the grasped surface. Comparisons to biological grasp strength highlights the stark inadequacy of the actuators, with the study examined in the previous chapter showing a mean average of 43.79 N for a 4-year-old child [16]. This discrepancy will only be overcome if small-scale actuators develop in such a way as to provide these heightened force outputs. Perhaps a more beneficial comparison is to look at the data for current prosthetic devices: 1.71 and 16.11 N. This puts the present device at approximately the median average. It is worth factoring in that these devices are all adult size and as such have slightly more flexibility in their approach to actuation; it also would seem fitting that adult prosthetics should have a higher grasp strength than their paediatric counterparts.

References

[1]   Vasluian E, Van Der Sluis CK, Van Essen AJ, *et al.* Birth prevalence for congenital limb defects in the northern Netherlands: A 30-year population-based study. BMC Musculoskeletal Disorders. 2013;14:323.

[2]   Dillingham TR, Pezzin LE, and MacKenzie EJ. Limb amputation and limb deficiency: Epidemiology and recent trends in the United States. Southern Medical Journal. 2002;95(8):875–883.

[3]   Egermann M, Kasten P, and Thomsen M. Myoelectric hand prostheses in very young children. International Orthopaedics. 2009;33(4):1101–1105.

[4]   Mano H, Fujiwara S, and Haga N. Adaptive behaviour and motor skills in children with upper limb deficiency. Prosthetics and Orthotics International. 2018;42(2):236–240.

[5]   Allami M, Mousavi B, Masoumi M, *et al.* A comprehensive musculoskeletal and peripheral nervous system assessment of war-related bilateral upper extremity amputees. Military Medical Research. 2016;3(1):1–8.

[6]   Postema S. Upper Limb Absence: Effects on Body Functions and Structures, Musculoskeletal Complaints, and Functional Capacity. REVALIDATIEGENEESKUNDE; 2017.

[7]   Meurs M, Maathuis CGB, Lucas C, Hadders-Algra M, and van der Sluis CK. Prescription of the first prosthesis and later use in children with congenital unilateral upper limb deficiency: A systematic review. Prosthetics and Orthotics International. 2006;30(2):165–173.

[8]   Scotland T and Galway H. A long-term review of children with congenital and acquired upper limb deficiency. The British Journal of Bone and Joint Surgery. 1983;65-B(3):346–349.

[9]   McGimpsey G and Bradford T. Limb Prosthetics Services and Devices: Critical Unmet Need: Market Analysis. Bioengineering Institute Center for Neuroprosthetics; 2017. p. 1–35.

[10] Walsh NE, and Walsh WS. Rehabilitation of landmine victims: The ultimate challenge. International Journal of Public Health 2003. 2003;81(9):665–670.

[11] Yoshikawa M, Sato R, Higashihara T, Ogasawara T, and Kawashima N. ReHand: Realistic electric prosthetic hand created with a 3D printer. In: 2015 37th Annual International Conference of the IEEE Engineering in Medicine and Biology Society (EMBC); 2015. p. 2470–2473.

[12] King M, Phillips B, Shively M, *et al.* Optimization of prosthetic hand manufacturing. In: 2015 IEEE Global Humanitarian Technology Conference (GHTC); 2015. p. 59–65.

[13]   Kargov A, Pylatiuk C, Martin J, Schulz S, and Döderlein L. A comparison of the grip force distribution in natural hands and in prosthetic hands. Disability and Rehabilitation. 2004;26(12):705–711.

[14]   Biddiss EA, and Chau TT. Upper limb prosthesis use and abandonment: A survey of the last 25 years. Prosthetics and Orthotics International. 2007;31(3):236–257.

[15]   Reaz MBI, Hussain MS, and Mohd-Yasin F. Techniques of EMG signal analysis: Detection, processing, classification and applications. Biological Procedures Online. 2006;8(1):11–35.

[16]   Muzumdar A. Powered Upper Limb Prostheses: Control, Implementation and Clinical Application. Berlin, Heidelberg: Springer-Verlag; 2004.

Chapter 11

The future of myoelectric prosthetics control

Kianoush Nazarpour[1]

11.1 Introduction

In the preceding ten chapters, we reviewed the state-of-the-art prosthetic control and shared several avenues for future work. We included research on the development of the hardware and software for prosthetics control and clinical evaluation.

The process of translating research advances in prosthetics control into real clinical gains for users of upper limb prostheses has been notoriously slow. Current clinical prostheses are mostly cosmetic or if active they are body controlled. The take-up of myoelectric devices is rare and the rate of device abandonment is significant. As such, the room for translation of advanced research method in a clinical setting is very tight. Overall, for a field which generates large numbers of academic papers, the clinical reality of the prevalence of non-users and rejectors of prostheses is both somewhat surprising and disappointing. Indeed, there remains significant evidence of dissatisfaction, with self-reported rejection rates of about 30%.

There are many potential underlying and explanatory factors. They include the mismatch between the rate of scientific and engineering innovation and clinical translation, lack of substantial clinical evidence that new methods would enhance the quality of life prosthesis users and the limited user involvement in the creation and testing of applicable solutions.

In this chapter, I will review these three factors. However, one must acknowledge that there are many other factors that fall outside the remit of this book. For example, the overall cost of the device, including the industrial research and development, manufacturing and testing, standardisation, marketing and commercial costs is one such factor. Together, these factors increase the ultimate price. Different local-level or national-level governmental policies and those by the insurance companies can also affect the affordability of the device.

[1]The University of Edinburgh, Edinburgh, UK

11.2   Are advanced prostheses fit for purpose?

As we indicated in the first chapter, myoelectric hands are controlled by using EMG signals that are generated on the contraction of remaining stump muscles. These signals are acquired by electrodes that are embedded within the socket and wired to the electronics in the prosthesis or in the cavity between the stump and the prosthesis. Research by Chadwell *et al.* [1] shows that even people with limb difference, who do not abandon their prosthesis, rely heavily on their intact limb. The reported reasons for limited prosthesis use or reject include the socket comfort and the weight of the whole device (socket and the prosthesis). Other key reasons are poor prosthesis control and limited functionality. As such the consensus among the researchers, clinicians and policymakers is that current prosthetics is not fit for purpose.

One of the key reasons that have slowed the development of myoelectric prostheses is the poor fidelity of the myoelectric sensors. Importantly, this is not because of the quality of the electronics. It is caused by the mechanical interaction between the sensor and the body. The EMG signal is sensitive to the position and orientation of the electrode with respect to the muscle fibres. There are no engineering or clinical methods to ensure the reliability of the electrode–skin contact during daily life. This uncertainty is worsened in the presence of the external forces that act on the socket. Also, internal forces such as those created by the movement of the arm can impact the quality of the signal negatively. Therefore, the key challenges are the identification and removal of the socket motion artefacts, which cause false activations of the prosthesis. Research is ongoing to address these problems by reducing the electrode–skin mechanical coupling [2]. Furthermore, smart machine-learning methods can estimate the likelihood of erroneous signal analysis and reject the control signal when the likelihood of the error is high.

Another challenge in verifying whether the current advanced prostheses meet the user needs is that use data, collected by the prosthetics industry, is not publicly available. This is expected and understandable from the commercial point of view; however, it does not help with the support in creating the evidence that is needed to convince the insurance companies and the national health system to underwrite the cost of advanced devices. However, this challenge does not stop at the commercial level. As we discussed in the second chapter, there are several review articles that attempt to identify the set of clinical outcome measures which should be used in the evaluation of the efficacy of these advanced devices [3,4]. However, there is still no consensus as to which outcome measures should be universally incorporated. A note of concern is that current methods are designed for testing within the boundaries of the clinic so they may not be generalisable to real-life everyday use. For instance, many tests such the SHAP are more concerned with the time it would take to achieve a task, e.g. pick and place objects. However, other factors such as the kinematics of reach and grasp, compensatory movements or postures are not taken into account quantitatively. These measures remain very much subjective. Another aspect may be that with the emergence of advanced prostheses that offer more than one active grip, e.g. via pattern recognition [5,6] or abstract control [7–9], there are no measures that quantify how the ability to switch between grips is utilised by the prosthesis users and whether that has a positive impact in the whole rehabilitation process and quality of life.

A move towards real-life outcome measures can create new opportunities to address the limitations with current approaches. Such real-world approaches to capturing and analysing data at scale are rapidly gaining popularity [10]. However, they introduce unanswered or open-ended questions in terms of data privacy and experiment integrity over unreliable communication networks and/or Internet. Research is still in infancy in these areas.

11.3   Novel technologies for prosthetic control

The rate of change in the area of prosthetic limbs is surprisingly slow. One can argue that the mechanical design of the prosthetic hands has improved significantly over the last decades. But the control of these devices in the clinical setting has not changed much. In the following, we review some of the technologies that have managed to get some space in the prosthetics industry or academia or have captured the imagination of the public.

11.3.1   Fast prototyping and 3D printing

Digital methods such as 3D scanning and printing have shown potential in research studies to facilitate the prototyping new test components in the process of developing advanced prosthetic hands.

The availability of 3D printers has led to the popular belief a wholly printed 3D hand and socket can replace the traditional manufacturing methods. Media have played an important role in engaging public emotively. Several commercial settings as well are trying to put forward this vision to the funding agencies and national health systems. However, the evidence is missing in terms of the robustness and the functionality of these devices. 3D-printed devices remain a commercial enterprise, particularly for children prosthetics. In the author's personal opinion, it is unlikely that 3D printing can replace traditional techniques in the short term unless controlled and randomised trials support the advantage of using these devices.

Notwithstanding the previous arguments, there may be other areas within the field of prosthetics that 3D printing can be more appropriate than the conventional methods – or at least offer an alternative paradigm. For example, the current clinical procedure to create a socket is a manual task. It is time-consuming and has low resolution. It requires a professional prosthetist [11,12]. The manual method of making prosthesis sockets has not changed significantly over the past decades. Several considerations have prevented the implementation of digital methods. Most companies providing digitally made sockets do so commercially. Therefore, published results are rare. But the studies that are published do not report the longevity or recall rate of digitally created devices.

Clinical evidence suggests that poor-fitting sockets can cause injuries to the remaining limb tissue and reduced device control [13,14]. Limb volume fluctuation, which is a key cause of poor socket fit [15], is influenced by many factors such as activity levels and diet [16]. Ideally, for every conspicuous change of limb volume, a new socket would be manufactured. However, this may not be feasible using traditional methods due to the time and manual labour involved. A digital workflow consisting 3D scanning, computer-aided design and 3D printing could help one to produce custom sockets more efficiently. Further research can determine whether 3D-printed sockets would be an appropriate option for long-term prosthesis control.

11.3.2 Implantable solutions

There is hope that the field of implantable microsystems neuroprosthetics could offer people with limb difference greatly increased functional recovery, both in terms of forward control of the device and also the feedback delivered to the nervous system. Despite significant progress, however, a considerable technological gap is there between our understanding of the fundamental sensorimotor neuroscience and the current state of the art in implantable microsystems that interact with the neuromuscular systems for the control of prosthetic hands. Examples of success from various laboratories are impressive but so far none of these technological innovations and amazing surgical methods and interventions are anywhere near widespread clinical translation. Research is fantastically active in several paths. These include the development of biomaterials and electrodes to readout muscle activity and/or interface bidirectionally with the peripheral nervous system, mathematical models to understand the neuromuscular codes and also the electronic technologies that could provide wirelessly enabled bidirectional interfacing. Such complementary research could revolutionise the fields of limb prosthetics and neural prosthetics in general. In addition, it can offer a new technological paradigm for interfacing with the autonomic nervous system, paving the way for future bioelectronic medicine.

11.3.3 New sensing modalities

The surface EMG signal suffers from poor spatial resolution. It is very challenging to target specific muscles even with high-density EMG sensors. Spatial resolution in the measurement of muscle activity can increase with invasive EMG sensors, which attach to muscles directly. For example, needle EMG recording is used clinically to diagnose muscle disease and offer a high spatial resolution. However, in addition to being painful, the penetration of the needle into the muscle disturbs the muscle structure and function. The application of wire/needle electrodes in prosthesis control has not gone beyond laboratory work. In chronic implants, such as for the control of motor prostheses, the interface between the metal contacts of the sensor and the muscle tissue changes over time, leading to infection and rejection by the body.

Research has investigated other sensory modalities. These include the use of inertial measurement of arm and skin movement [6,17–20]. Specifically, the latter has been referred to as sensing the accelerometry of the skin movement because of muscle activity, mechanomyography or force myography. Despite these being put in a single category, we admit that there are differences between these methods.

Another long-standing myography method is A-mode ultrasound scanning of the muscle activity via one or more ultrasound probes. This is also called sonomyography. This approach has proved very successful in imaging muscle activity. However, it has not moved beyond laboratory investigation due to the requirement of the gel and the level of energy consumption that is significantly more than what can be supplied by the current batteries in prosthetic solutions.

In the fourth chapter of this book, we introduced magnetomyography (MMG) [21–24] as an alternative method to measure muscle activity. MMG has the potential to address both limitations of the EMG method:

1.   The magnetic field generated by muscle activity has the same temporal resolution as the EMG signal but offers significantly higher spatial resolution.
2.   It does not require electric contacts for recording and hence, the sensor can be fully encapsulated with a biocompatible material before implantation, minimising the risk of infection.

Recently, tunneling magnetoresistive sensors [25] and optimally pumped magnetometers [26] have been used to record MMG signals.

A totally different sensory modality, which we did not cover in this book, is the use of artificial vision. The vision-augmented prosthesis control for semi-autonomous grasp identification has been proposed with varying success [27–30].

All of these alternative sensing modalities are in the early stages of development and verification. But they have huge potential in replacing the EMG signal and providing a significant step-change in the way the muscle activity is detected. A most desirable solution is to be able to sense muscle activity with a high spatiotemporal resolution at minimal energy and computational cost.

11.4   User needs

Academic collaboration with external stakeholders, including users of prosthetic devices, can create impact by focusing on identified user needs. One approach to this collaboration is co-creation, which is a collaborative process in which knowledge is generated by academics working alongside other stakeholders throughout the research process [31]. Co-creation engages with stakeholders from the onset of a research study: from framing initial research questions to the dissemination of results. In the United Kingdom, this approach has been championed by the National Institute for Health Research since 1996.

Engineering and medical advancement in academia are predominately laboratory-based. However, there is evidence that laboratory-used metrics and findings are not always consistent with clinical outcomes. Therefore, there is a movement towards testing devices and systems within people's home environment in order to enable clinical translation. For this to be successful, academia might be required to work with different organisations, such as user groups, healthcare providers, policymakers, industry specialists and medical charities, in a collaborative manner.

Involvement of users throughout the research, development and implementation phases of projects can lead to a decline in the rate of prosthesis abandonment. There is potential for this to be achieved through the adoption of co-creation, by combining co-advocacy, co-production and development and co-governance.

References

[1] Chadwell A, Kenney L, Granat MH, *et al.* Upper limb activity in myoelectric prosthesis users is biased towards the intact limb and appears unrelated to goal-directed task performance. Scientific Reports. 2018;8(1):11084.

[2] Jabran A, Tomanec F, Kenney L, *et al.* Assessment of adjustable electrode housing device for transradial myoelectric prostheses. In: Trent International Prosthetics Symposium. Salford, UK; 2019. p. 1.

[3] World Health Organisation. ICF International Classification of Functioning, Disability and Health. [World Health Organisation Report]; 2001.

[4] World Health Organisation. Towards a Common Language for Functioning, Disability and Health: ICF Beginner's Guide. [World Health Organisation Report]; 2002.

[5] Farina D, Jiang N, Rehbaum H, *et al.* The extraction of neural information from the surface EMG for the control of upper-limb prostheses: emerging avenues and challenges. IEEE Transactions on Neural Systems and Rehabilitation Engineering. 2014;22(4):797–809.

[6] Krasoulis A, Vijayakumar S, and Nazarpour K. Multi-grip classification-based prosthesis control with two EMG-IMU sensors. IEEE Transactions on Neural Systems and Rehabilitation Engineering. 2020;28(2):508–518.

[7] Pistohl T, Cipriani C, Jackson A, and Nazarpour K. Abstract and proportional myoelectric control for multi-fingered hand prostheses. Annals of Biomedical Engineering. 2013;41(12):2687–2698.

[8] Antuvan CW, Ison M, and Artemiadis P. Embedded human control of robots using myoelectric interfaces. IEEE Transactions on Neural Systems and Rehabilitation Engineering. 2014;22(4):820–827.

[9] Dyson M, Barnes J, and Nazarpour K. Myoelectric control with abstract decoders. Journal of Neural Engineering. 2018;15(5):056003.

[10] Ottenbacher KJ, Graham JE, and Fisher SR. Data science in physical medicine and rehabilitation: opportunities and challenges. Physical Medicine and Rehabilitation Clinics of North America. 2019;30(2):459–471. Available from: https://www.ncbi.nlm.nih.gov/pubmed/30954159.

[11] Steer JW, Grudniewski PA, Browne M, Worsley PR, Sobey AJ, and Dickinson AS. Predictive prosthetic socket design: Part 2—Generating person-specific candidate designs using multi-objective genetic algorithms. Biomechanics and Modeling in Mechanobiology. 2020;19:1347–1360

[12] Davies R and Russell D. Vacuum formed thermoplastic sockets for prostheses. In: Disability. London, UK: Palgrave Macmillan; 1979. p. 385–390.

[13] Chadwell A, Kenney L, Thies S, Galpin A, and Head J. The reality of myoelectric prostheses: Understanding what makes these devices difficult for some users to control. Frontiers in Neurorobotics. 2016;10:7.

[14] Wernke MM, Schroeder RM, Haynes ML, Nolt LL, Albury AW, and Colvin JM. Progress toward optimizing prosthetic socket fit and suspension using elevated vacuum to promote residual limb health. Advances in Wound Care. 2017;6(7):233–239.

[15] Sanders JE, Harrison DS, Allyn KJ, and Myers TR. Clinical utility of in-socket residual limb volume change measurement: case study results. Prosthetics and Orthotics International. 2009;33(4):378–390.

[16] Sanders JE and Fatone S. Residual limb volume change: systematic review of measurement and management. Journal of Rehabilitation Research and Development. 2011;48(8):949.

[17] Krasoulis A, Vijayakumar S, and Nazarpour K. Evaluation of regression methods for the continuous decoding of finger movement from surface EMG and accelerometry. In: Proc. IEEE/EMBS Int. Conf. Neur. Eng.; 2015. p. 631–634.

[18] Krasoulis A, Kyranou I, Erden MS, Nazarpour K, and Vijayakumar S. Improved prosthetic hand control with concurrent use of myoelectric and inertial measurements. Journal of NeuroEngineering and Rehabilitation. 2017;14(1):71.

[19] Radmand A, Scheme E, and Englehart K. On the suitability of integrating accelerometry data with electromyography signals for resolving the effect of changes in limb position during dynamic limb movement. Journal of Prosthetics and Orthotics. 2014;26(4):185–193.

[20] Khushaba RN, Al-Timemy A, Kodagoda S, and Nazarpour K. Combined influence of forearm orientation and muscular contraction on EMG pattern recognition. Expert Systems with Applications. 2016;61:154–161.

[21] Heidari H, Zuo S, Krasoulis A, and Nazarpour K. CMOS magnetic sensors for wearable magnetomyography. In: 40th International Conference of the IEEE Engineering in Medicine and Biology Society; 2018. p. 2116–2119.

[22] Zuo S, Nazarpour K, and Heidari H. Device modeling of MgO-barrier tunneling magnetoresistors for hybrid spintronic-CMOS. IEEE Electron Device Letters. 2018;39(11):1784–1787.

[23] Zuo S, Fan H, Nazarpour K, and Heidari H. A CMOS analog front-end for tunnelling magnetoresistive spintronic sensing systems. In: 2019 IEEE International Symposium on Circuits and Systems (ISCAS); 2019. p. 1–5.

[24] Zuo S, Nazarpour K, Böhnert T, Ferreira R, and Heidari H. Integrated pico-tesla resolution magnetoresistive sensors for miniaturised magnetomyography. In: 42nd Annual International Conference of the IEEE Engineering in Medicine and Biology Society (EMBC); 2020. p. 1–5.

[25] Zuo S, Heidari H, Farina D, and Nazarpour K. Miniaturized Magnetic Sensors for Implantable Magnetomyography. Advanced Materials Technologies; 2020. p. 2000185.

[26]   Broser PJ, Knappe S, Kajal DS, *et al.* Optically pumped magnetometers for magneto-myography to study the innervation of the hand. IEEE Transactions on Neural Systems and Rehabilitation Engineering. 2018;26(11):2226–2230.

[27]   Došen S and Popović DB. Transradial prosthesis: artificial vision for control of prehension. Artificial Organs. 2011;35(1):37–48.

[28]   Markovic M, Dosen S, Cipriani C, Popovic D, and Farina D. Stereovision and augmented reality for closed-loop control of grasping in hand prostheses. Journal of Neural Engineering. 2014;11(4):046001.

[29]   Ghazaei G, Alameer A, Degenaar P, Morgan G, and Nazarpour K. An exploratory study on the use of convolutional neural networks for object grasp classification. In: Proc. 2nd IET Int. Conf. Intell. Signal Process.; 2015. p. 5.

[30]   Ghazaei G, Alameer A, Degenaar P, Morgan G, and Nazarpour K. Deep learning-based artificial vision for grasp classification in myoelectric hands. Journal of Neural Engineering. 2017;14(3):036025.

[31]   Jones H, Supan S, and Nazarpour K. The future of prosthetics: a user perspective. In: Trent International Prosthetics Symposium. Salford, UK; 2019. p. 1.

Index

www.ingramcontent.com/pod-product-compliance
Lightning Source LLC
Chambersburg PA
CBHW050516190326
41458CB00005B/1559